MENTAL HEALTH IN CRISIS

SAGE SWIFTS

In 1976 SAGE published a series of short 'university papers', which led to the publication of the QASS series (or the 'little green books' as they became known to researchers). More than 40 years since the release of the first 'little green book', SAGE is delighted to offer a new series of swift, short and topical pieces in the ever-growing digital environment.

SAGE *Swifts* offer authors a new channel for academic research with the freedom to deliver work outside the conventional length of journal articles. The series aims to give authors speedy access to academic audiences through digital first publication, space to explore ideas thoroughly, yet at a length which can be readily digested, and the quality stamp and reassurance of peer-review.

MENTAL HEALTH IN CRISIS

JOEL VOS,
RON ROBERTS
JAMES DAVIES

SAGE SWIFTS

SAGE

Los Angeles | London | New Delhi
Singapore | Washington DC | Melbourne

SAGE

Los Angeles | London | New Delhi
Singapore | Washington DC | Melbourne

SAGE Publications Ltd
1 Oliver's Yard
55 City Road
London EC1Y 1SP

SAGE Publications Inc.
2455 Teller Road
Thousand Oaks, California 91320

SAGE Publications India Pvt Ltd
B 1/I 1 Mohan Cooperative Industrial Area
Mathura Road
New Delhi 110 044

SAGE Publications Asia-Pacific Pte Ltd
3 Church Street
#10-04 Samsung Hub
Singapore 049483

Editor: Susannah Trefgarne
Assistant editor: Talulah Hall
Production editor: Rachel Burrows
Copyeditor: Solveig Gardner Servian
Proofreader: David Hemsley
Indexer: David Rudeforth
Marketing manager: Samantha Glorioso
Cover design: Sheila Tong
Typeset by: C&M Digitals (P) Ltd, Chennai, India

First published 2019

Library of Congress Control Number: 2019930847

British Library Cataloguing in Publication data

A catalogue record for this book is available from the British Library

ISBN 978-1-5264-9220-3
ISBN 978-1-5264-9258-6 (web PDF)

CONTENTS

INTRODUCTION

Joel Vos & Ron Roberts

> Times of crisis, of disruption or constructive change, are not only predictable, but desirable. They mean growth. Taking a new step, uttering a new word, is what people fear most.
>
> Dostoyevksi

We live in an age of crises. Once infallible banks and corporations have been shaken to their foundations and have brought uncertainty into the lives of many. Our unrelenting desire for a comfortable life has given rise to pollution, melting polar ice-caps, incessant war and mass starvation. Austerity measures and benefit cuts have hit many and made food banks a normal sight in wealthy societies. Escalating international conflicts have sent numerous families into a refugees' no-man's land. While some find solace in supporting populist politics, others see their nightmares realised with the rise of the political alt-right and authoritarian leaders striding the world stage. The multiple crises pervading the global stage are entangled – economic instability, ethnic conflict, authoritarianism and Brexit – creating a tide of instability which shows no signs of abating.

This book argues the unfolding mental health crises we see are related to wider social upheavals. The global crises are mirrored in personal crises. How could this be otherwise? The Holocaust survivor Viktor Frankl believed a personal crisis can be a normal response to an abnormal situation. From this perspective, it is surprising how many remain sane and continue in their daily routines apparently untroubled. Such persistence however, with its oft accompanying denial and avoidance, is not necessarily a sign of well-being.

The crisis in mental health has two faces. On the one hand, we see people struggling with mental health problems – a response to financial uncertainty, benefit cuts or discrimination. On the other hand, there is a crisis in the way individuals with mental health problems are understood and treated. This book will show how, instead of listening to the lived experience of individuals, ostensible mental health experts impose diagnostic models and interventions which reflect the interests of financial lobbyists more than the needs of clients. Thus, we stare into a crisis in mental health and a crisis in mental health care, both embedded in a world facing multiple crises.

Being-in-crisis does not exclude hope. For the Ancient Greek physicians, *krisis* signified a critical point of change, for better or worse, in the health of the patient. So there is an opportunity for recovery, that we can find a meaningful and satisfying way of living despite the challenges we face. Although this book is principally concerned with the crises in mental health, we keep one eye on prospective solutions. The mental health crisis gives us an opportunity to take stock, reflect and move towards a different future – one with better mental health and mental health care and a society predicated on different values. This critical yet optimistic spirit pervaded the lectures, workshops and music events of the charity Punk4MentalHealth that inspired the birth of this book in Spring 2017.

Each of the following chapters describe a different crisis in mental health or society. The first shows how societal problems are often regarded and treated as individual problems. Fortunately, mental health care is increasingly shifting attention to the client's socio-economic context, and offering care more often in the community than the isolation of the hospital. Following this we examine how austerity measures and benefit cuts from governments have affected citizens' mental well-being, and particularly poorer educated, female, black and gay individuals. Subsequent chapters on the financial, biomedical and drugs crises in mental health address how the care system is often organised to primarily benefit stakeholders with professional or financial interests. We note a clear crisis in the system of assigning psychiatric diagnoses, the empirical foundations of which are highly questionable. We argue the system disadvantages individuals, conferring both stigma and a dubious basis for treatment. We then progress to deeper sociological and philosophical layers which contemplate how the capitalist system influences mental health, particularly the organisation of the mental health care system. The final chapters of the book explore alternatives for the crises we have documented.

While writing this book, we considered using the terms 'alternative' or 'critical' in the title as these terms are frequently used interchangeably. However, we quickly realised some of the perspectives discussed here, framed as 'alternative' or 'critical', could better be considered mainstream owing to the changes afoot. These perspectives are based on systematic empirical evidence and not on esoteric hypothetical philosophies. Asking questions about the empirical foundations of mental health is not alternative but a quintessential scientific activity that professionals could engage in. One aspect of the crisis in mental health is that strong paradigmatic stories in the field label as 'outcasts' any approach 'deviating' from them. We wish to reveal the limitations of these paradigms, and reveal options beyond the disintegrating status quo. We believe there is no need for mental health to be in the crisis it now is, so long as individuals are supported adequately by their governments and those professionally charged with their care. To add weight to the voices in this book and to show them as far from uncommon, we include below a letter published in the *Independent* on 4 November 2017 (reproduced with permission) from the presidents of all principal mental health bodies in the UK.

> *We, leading mental health bodies in the UK, are calling on the government to take immediate action to address the rising levels of mental ill-health.*
>
> *The Government must increase investment in mental health services and ring-fence the mental health budget, ahead of the Autumn Budget. The focus must also be on investing upstream to prevent mental health problems from developing and escalating into crisis.*
>
> *Without this action, it will not be possible to absorb the spiralling costs of services associated with providing the best care and support.*
>
> *The majority of children and adults with mental health issues are unable to get the help they need – nor will they get it any time soon.*
>
> *With a government target for just 25 per cent of adults with mental health issues to access talking therapies by 2020, parity of esteem remains very unlikely.*
>
> *For children the situation is not much better, the 2020 mental health access target of just 35 per cent still leaves the remaining 65 per cent locked out of services.*
>
> *The Government has said repeatedly that it's investing £1bn extra in mental health services per year, but that money falls short of what is needed, and often isn't reaching the front line.*

Freedom of Information requests have shown that over half of Clinical Commissioning Groups (CCGs) plan to reduce the proportion of their budget they spend on mental health for 2016–17.

We cannot go on with such unambitious targets, or simply accept a situation where promises of extra funding don't actually materialise at the front line.

If the Government is actually to deliver parity of esteem, the Chancellor needs to invest in and ring-fence the mental health budget to ensure any money promised genuinely reaches those it is intended to help. The crisis is here, the crisis is now.

Yours sincerely,

Sarah Niblock, Chief Executive, UK Council for Psychotherapy

Jenny Edwards CBE, CEO, Mental Health Foundation

Sarah Brennan OBE, CEO, Young Minds

Tom Quinn, director of external affairs, B-EAT

Piers Watson, chair, OCD Action

Gary Fereday, CEO, British Psychoanalytic Council

Dr Hadyn Williams, chief executive, British Association for Counselling and Psychotherapy

Heather Stewart, chair, Association Child Psychotherapists

Nicola Gale, president, British Psychological Society

Catherine Roche, chief executive, Place2Be

Vicky Parkinson, CEO, National Counselling Society

Andrew Balfour, CEO, Tavistock Relationships

1

COMMUNITY CRISIS

Joel Vos

> Modern man no longer communicates with the madman ... There is no common language ... The language of psychiatry, which is a monologue by reason about madness, could only have come into existence in such a silence.
>
> Foucault, 2003: 5

THE COPERNICAN REVOLUTION IN MENTAL HEALTH CARE

In modern history, individuals with mental health problems have often occupied a difficult place in their communities (Foucault, 2003). This chapter describes the complex relationship between individuals with mental health problems and society. We will argue that a Copernican revolution is in our midst, with individuals less likely to be treated as pariahs against whom society should be protected. Instead, it is society which is now seen as oppressive and stigmatising and individuals more often supported within their communities. The role of mental health care is transforming from individual-oriented to social-context-oriented care. However, structural injustices persist.

The history of individuals with mental health problems opens with a dark chapter. Until the late European Middle Ages, people lived their lives according to the expectations of their social context – family, church and landlords. When their well-being prevented them fulfilling expected roles, their lives were deemed meaningless (Vos, 2018). Mental health problems were seen as moral issues which prevented individuals realising their pre-ordained station in the socio-cosmic-divine order. Problematic behaviours were deemed 'evil' and individuals designated as sources of malign contagion became outcasts, sent away to colonies or under due legal process burned at the stake. The 'lucky' were 'taken care of' in religious madhouses, such as Bethlem, which was set up to care for patients in London in 1377.

The medical profession began to conceptualise mental health problems as physical afflictions from the 17th century onwards, establishing numerous 'madhouses' in England. Following the Lunacy/Lunatics Act 1845, a network of country asylums was built. Little treatment existed in these, which were effectively 'warehouses for the unwanted' (Glasby & Tew, 2015: 29). Bethlam became a tourist attraction, with over 100,000 annual visitors seeing the patients in cages. Many asylum doctors argued that mental vulnerability was caused by tainted genes, a then common view. During the 19th century, doctors began experimenting with 'cures' – lobotomy, electro-convulsive therapy, drugs – which owed more to trial-and-error than scientific evidence.

At the same time, philosophers developed the idea that our psychological experiences are not necessarily biophysical in origin but the result of our ways of reasoning and psychological associations. At the end of the 19th century, Freud instigated the 'talking cure' to help individuals. Instead of the asylum, patients saw him in his home. Like his contemporaries, Freud focused on the individual not the social context. Initially he considered clients had developed neuroses because of traumatic childhood experiences such as incest. Later however, he recanted, arguing that so many reported similar experiences that not all of them could be real. He subsequently developed his theory of the Oedipus complex, holding that patients' reports of abuse were incest fantasies.

Freud's theories contributed to the individualisation and psychologisation of real-life experiences, a common tendency within the nascent discipline of psychology. Skinner and Pavlov, in turn, demonstrated how animals and people create psychological associations, for example between a bell ringing and the delivery of food when both occur at the same time. The sound of the bell develops the meaning of 'food' for the animal, although this does not objectively indicate food. In this behaviourist paradigm, mental health problems are seen as the result of conditioning and reinforcement. Behaviour therapy came to focus on analysing individual association patterns and learning new behaviour.

In their early versions, all three paradigms – medical, psychodynamic and behaviourist – located the cause and solution of mental health problems in the individual. This assumption has long determined the diagnosis and treatment of 'mentally-ill patients'. Mental health services were designed to cure individual pathologies, attention rarely being given to clients' subjective experiences as their views were considered pathological and irrelevant. Because of this, patients were disbelieved when they spoke about abuse in their family, community, church or hospital. Criticisms about mistreatment in psychiatric clinics also seldom reached a general audience, enabling mistreatment to continue. As Smail (1987: 69) argues, such beliefs about 'the reasons for our conduct' are 'designed to repress'; we then 'come to feel' personally responsible 'for social injustices' perpetuated 'beyond the reach of our awareness'.

COMMUNITY PSYCHOLOGY

Influenced by the First World War, Freud returned to the idea that the wider context could influence mental health. Jungian analysis, which emphasised universal archetypical experiences, and philosophical analysis of our shared existential struggles, added to the growing interest in the common conditions of our lives. 'Shell shock' in soldiers returning from the front came to be seen as unrelated to one's biological constitution or internal psychodynamics. Recognition of an external reality which influences people's mental health, and that individuals shared common experiences, meant they were not completely to blame for their plight.

The British Mental Treatment Act 1930 supported out-patient treatment for mental health problems, funded by local authorities. The birth of the British National Health Service (NHS) in 1948 saw mental health services become more widely available, albeit underfunded. Financially and socially, this system appeared unsustainable, so by the late 1950s, the idea of treating patients in the community rather than hospitals began to grow. As asylums began closing psychotherapy clinics opened, meaning individuals received help from day care, social work support and sheltered employment. This deinstitutionalisation was due to a combination of factors: the development of new pharmaceutical and psychotherapeutic treatments which didn't require hospitalisation; poor conditions in asylums; greater acceptance of individuals with mental health problems; and lack of funding. However, one of the most important factors was a different view on mental health and care – that individuals were not always to blame for their problems.

A critical psychiatry movement emerged, and films such as *One Flew Over the Cuckoo's Nest* (1975) brought the power dynamics in psychiatric settings to public attention. Ronnie Laing, who listened and empathised with his patients in order to understand the logic of their experiences, was a significant figure in this movement, which spread beyond the UK. Franz Fanon, Paolo Friere and Steve Biko directed attention to the political context. So the idea evolved that people's mental health could be understood within a wider social framework. During the 1970s, critical psychology emerged, influenced by the Frankfurt School and post-structuralism. The 1980s saw the emergence of community psychology in Latin America, situating the community as the focal point of psychological action.

These developments signalled a movement away from individuals toward the wider community, one seen as efficient, beneficial for mental health and empowering. This chapter will describe the shifts in thinking that underlay this transformation.

INDIVIDUALS-IN-CONTEXT

The 'mentally ill' were traditionally seen as victims of defective biology, conflicted psychodynamic drives or maladaptive learned behaviour. The social context was reduced to an 'object' or 'stimulus' that the individual responds to. However, theoretical developments in psychodynamics and behaviourism acknowledged the context of the individual as a primary cause of problems. Object-relation theorists, such as Klein and Winnicott, and attachment theorists such as Bowlby and Ainsworth, argued that individuals develop fundamental psychological patterns, such as insecure attachment, in response to early experiences. Behaviourists argued that operant conditioning (by reinforcement or punishment) could account for aberrant behaviour while others suggested a role for dysfunctional family dynamics.

Though the focus widened from the individual to their immediate social context, this did not imply that political struggles and socio-economic circumstances were seen as potential causes of problem behaviour. Ironically, numerous accounts exist of governments using mental health care to manipulate political opponents, branding them 'mentally ill' and exposing them to invasive 'treatments' such as electroconvulsive therapy (ECT). The American Central Intelligence Agency (CIA), for example, developed an instructional manual of how to mentally torture political opponents, whilst in the USSR dissidents were sent to asylums (Klein, 2007). Under the McCarthy regime in the US, supposed communists were also subjected to involuntary psychiatric treatments. Mental health care thus functioned as a domain of political repression. When the US army intervened in Chile, Brazil and

Iraq, they brought with them numerous psychiatrists and other 'behavioural science experts' as members of their strategic force.

Paulo Freire (1970) was among the first to expose the political use of mental health. Though his work focused primarily on education, it has been extensively applied in mental health care. Freire considered all education either indoctrinates individuals into conformity or else becomes a practice of freedom enabling people to deal critically with their reality. Similar voices were heard in colonial countries, such as Algeria. The psychiatrist Franz Fanon (1952/1967) describes how black people were perceived as lesser beings by white people, and how this perception created feelings of insecurity and inferiority in black individuals. Fanon's work inspired Steve Biko in the anti-apartheid struggle in South Africa and Malcolm X in the American civil rights movement. Their work showed how black people, ethnic minority groups and those without socio-political power are oppressed, not only in the practical/physical domain but also the psychological. Referring to such developments, Sedgwick (1982) concluded that mental health must be seen through a political lens, and appealed for collective responsibility for the care of people with mental health problems.

These authors and activists effectively laid the foundations for critical community psychology to examine the dominant narratives in psychology, and reveal how political and socio-economic circumstances shape both individual well-being and social justice (Kagan et al., 2011), and thus that the intra-personal, inter-personal and political-ideological domains cannot be clearly separated (Orford, 2008). They have since argued that to improve mental health, people's politico-socio-economic circumstances should be enhanced, via individual empowerment, community action and mental health advocacy. An impressive body of research has strengthened their arguments.

FROM NATURE–NURTURE TO ECOLOGICAL PSYCHOLOGY

In the 1980s–1990s, the nature–nurture debate dominated mental health discourse. This concerned the respective contributions of genetic inheritance and upbringing/environment to mental health. The debate was often couched in Manichean terms, suggesting only one side could be right. Recent research suggests a more complex model involving the combined influence of genes, the physical and social environment, lifestyle and coping.

There is evidence to link genetic variations with diagnoses of schizophrenia (Tsuang et al., 1999), autism (Happé & Ronald, 2008) and mood disorders (Jacobson & Cryan, 2007). Although mental health problems may have biological correlates, they do not necessarily stem from them (Harré, 2002). Other physical factors are also influential. Having older parents or experiencing problems during pregnancy or birth increases the risk of developing schizophrenia (Matheson, et al., 2011), although some consider the risks may only impact those with specific genetic vulnerabilities. Particular genes may be 'switched on' in the presence of specific life events; for example, one genetic polymorphism is associated with depression later in life only when the individual has also experienced severe childhood trauma (Lok et al., 2013).

So psychological context shapes mental health, either alone or in interaction with biological factors. Philosophers have contemplated how societal trends can influence mental health; the present dystopia, characterised by widespread nihilism, narcissism and consumerism can influence how individuals develop (Levin, 1987). We will discuss later how social oppression has been linked with mental health problems. Numerous studies show psychosis and social disadvantage are correlated, leading to the hypothesis that powerlessness and subordination have biological and psychological consequences. Furthermore, the experience of blame or stigma may contribute to mental health problems. While situational and cultural circumstances may operate on a prior genetic vulnerability, research suggests that social, physical and economic circumstances influence mental health directly, with no underlying genetic vulnerability.

In addition to the factors described above, an individual's lifestyle influences mental well-being. Smoking marijuana for instance increases risk of psychosis, whilst other drugs – including prescribed – may also create structural changes in the brain. What the long-term effects of these are remains unclear (Moncrieff, 2009). Researchers have also shown how individuals can experience an inner freedom and flexibility to cope in beneficial ways with difficult life situations. Similarly, people's coping styles are important (Vos, 2018). In summary, mental health problems develop as a consequence of a complex combination and interaction of factors. This carries implications for interventions in different domains.

Fortunately, research shows that the brain is more flexible than previously thought. Later life experiences and life choices may also be critical to good mental health. Research shows that one's personality significantly changes over the life course and that interventions, such as psychotherapy, can also change personality (Roberts et al., 2017). This research shows that individual and community mental health interventions have great potential.

Community psychologists have criticised mental health services for their narrow focus on the individual. For instance, many psychotherapeutic approaches address the individual's *experience* of their life situation, although that situation may be unjust and a primary cause of problems. Psychotherapy individualises distress and ignores the complex real world in which we live (Smail, 2005). Mental health care systems have thereby been criticised for failing in their promise of progressive humanism (Pilgrim, 1997). Neglecting the wider parameters of human struggle, the psy-professions have intensified the gaze on individuals. The consequent self-blaming that can occur in psychotherapy can act as an additional burden.

FROM UNIVERSAL LAWS TO DIVERSITY

Elsewhere, we describe the unreliable scientific foundations of psychiatric diagnosis and note the influence of political lobbies on their development (Davies, 2013). Despite this, treatment is often based on such diagnoses and access to care is contingent on them. This diagnostic model also determines whether individuals will be recipients of coercive mental health care.

In recent decades, the universality of mental health categories has come under increasing fire. Phenomenologists argue that a mental health disorder is not an objective entity, such as a fever that can be reliably physically assessed. Mental health problems concern the way someone relates to their experiences and the situations they encounter. For example, when depressed you do not only see the world and others negatively, you feel and think negatively about yourself and your mental health, thereby affecting how you cope. As a result of this researchers have investigated 'illness perception', with different individuals having different ideas about mental health problems such as schizophrenia (Lobban et al., 2005). With different ideas about what it means to have a condition, people attribute their problems to different causes, have different ideas about its likely course and impact on their life, and what interventions may be appropriate. This subjective perception is often ignored in standardised mental health care. Humanistic and existential therapists reject the universality of diagnosis, and pay specific attention to individuals' unique experiences.

There is increasing interest in mental health models in non-western peoples. The ways in which cultures differ from each other may have great relevance to perceptions of mental health, their causes and their treatments (Cox, 2018). Not only cultural differences influence ideas about mental health, but also subcultures (e.g. punks and hip-hoppers). We must be careful, however; cultural/subcultural identity and sense of self are not monoliths with one specific perception of mental health; individuals often experience different 'selves' in different contexts. This implies that no one-size-fits-all assessment of problems and solutions is adequate, and that listening, empathy and tailoring are core skills for practitioners. Research throughout the UK shows that using standardised treatment manuals is not more effective than tailored person-centred care (Truijens et al., 2018). Consequently, there is a movement away from universal assumptions towards embracing a diversity of voices in mental health. Unfortunately, NHS services remain dominantly focused on standardised interventions.

FROM INDIVIDUAL CURE TO SOCIAL RECOVERY

The medical model suggests that mental health problems can be 'cured' on the basis of diagnosed psychopathology. Available data provides little support for this. Meta-analyses suggest that most pharmaceutical treatments produce only modest improvements, whereas psychotherapy and counselling lead to modest to large improvements (Lambert, 2013). These studies also show that effects decrease over time and around one-third of patients relapse. In comparison, *most* clients with severe mental health problems who stop using pharmaceutical drugs relapse, suggesting they do not undergo a structural 'cure' unlike clients who can live well after psychotherapy. There is also considerable variation and good reason to believe that a treatment does not have the same effect on every individual in a given situation.

The figures given focus only on improvement in relation to a formal psychiatric diagnosis. Many clients, when asked what type of improvement they desire, indicate that they want to learn how to live a meaningful and satisfying life – as defined by themselves – despite any ongoing problems (Vos, 2018). This is particularly the case for those with severe problems (Andresen et al., 2011). The focus on improvement in psychiatric terms may be irrelevant to clients who want to be in control of their lives, able to live a full normal daily life in their own community. Research is positive about this. There is good evidence (392 trials involving 28,808 participants) that psychological therapies produce a large improvement in people's ability to live a meaningful life (Vos, 2018).

This focus on recovery rather than cure has been considered in several western countries. It implies a dramatic shift in the role of the mental health practitioner, from being an authority who imposes their opinion on clients to being an empathic listener and facilitator. This recovery approach often means clients are supported in their community – in developing positive social relationships and engaging in employment or voluntary work. On a practical level, the policy has led to the development of recovery colleges where clients can learn life skills. However, development of the approach has been hindered by organisational resistance. The Mental Health Act 2007 and subsequent policies have once again focused on the paternalistic role and coercive power of health professionals (Glasby & Tew, 2015).

POWER STRUCTURES AND EMPOWERMENT

During the 1960s–1970s, an international movement evolved, critical of traditional medical approaches to mental health. Protagonists in this so-called anti-psychiatry movement were inspired by wider political activism. Foucault (2002) described how modern medicine dehumanised individuals with mental health problems. He describes how the 'medical gaze' separates an objective medical problem from a person's subjective experience and identity. In asylums and madhouses, doctors reduced the lived experience of patients to biological phenomena which could be medically 'attacked'. Due to this separation between symptoms and patient, the patient no longer owned their problems which now belonged to medicine, with all its associated interests, dynamics and coercive possibilities. The patient had become 'subject' to the machinations of medical doctors who sought compliance with societal expectations of 'sane behaviour'.

Numerous forms of discipline became the focus of Foucault's later work (2012), addressing how individuals are continuously subject to the strategic ploys of institutional actors (e.g. in mental health clinics and schools), manipulated to conform to socially prescribed roles. This manipulation can be explicit and external or implicit and internal, leading individuals to be continuously self-critical and to feel guilt or shame when they do not fit their expected role. In this way, oppression and psychological repression go hand in hand (Deleuze & Guattari, 2004). Social oppression begins early in the family, with parents trying to control children's desires. This leads the children to repress parts of themselves, leading to later problems. Thus, both the aetiology and the psychiatric treatment of mental health problems are interwoven with societal forces of power and manipulation.

This critical philosophy led some psychiatrists to experiment with alternative forms of care. From listening to clients' stories, Laing considered the source of distress to lie in the urban home and institutions in which selves are forged, relocating irrationality from the mental health patient to the society (Laing, 1990). Such thinking has influenced practitioners worldwide. For example, person-centred and existential psychotherapists do not follow the traditional pattern of psychiatric labelling and imposing their ideas on clients. They prefer to work on building positive relationships with clients, to understand them and help with their subjective needs. Therapists inform clients explicitly what they can do, and negotiate the aims and method of the sessions (Cantwell et al., 2015). A core competence for this is reflexivity, as therapists aim for awareness of potential power differences in the therapeutic relationship. Freire (1970) called this 'conscientisation': developing a critical understanding of themselves and their reality, and understanding the social dynamics of how this reality has come into being. On this basis possibilities for action can be developed. Empowerment means that practitioners and community workers help individuals gain control over their lives, develop critical awareness of the socio-political environment and enhance democratic participation in communities. This goes beyond helping individuals develop psychological resources to cope with their life circumstances. Mental health care here becomes a tool for empowerment beyond the therapy room.

Many training schools in critical and existential-humanistic approaches have developed, such as the Philadelphia Association, the New School of Psychotherapy and Counselling (NSPC), and the Metanoia Institute in London. Many clinics work explicitly from a humanistic perspective. In Soteria clinics, patients and staff are seen as equals. The Hearing Voices Network (HVN) is another example where the focus lies on the social connections and recovery of clients, and normalising their experiences of extraordinary experiences such as hearing, seeing or feeling things that others cannot. Research shows that these approaches are effective in helping individuals to live a meaningful life and reducing their psychopathological symptoms (Vos et al., 2015; Elliott et al., 2013). Nationwide outcome monitoring has shown that these humanistic therapies are no less effective than others (Barkham & Saxon, 2018). Despite this evidence, UK guidelines have yet to include humanistic therapies as standard.

DISCUSSION

Research shows that mental health experiences result from a complex combination and interaction of factors, some of which are individual but most of which are social. Simultaneously, mental health care is being increasingly provided in the community, and problems increasingly understood in their larger social context. Unfortunately, many groups continue to experience stigmatisation and discrimination.

It is important that practitioners and policy makers are educated in the complex integrative framework of mental health, and are made aware of the injustices and pains that result from an individual-focused approach. This chapter argues that individual mental health may be shaped by the deleterious effects of structural power imbalances in society. Policy makers should therefore aim to address socio-economic inequalities, and include the voices of service users (Lustig, 2012).

This chapter has also shown the importance of delivering non-stigmatising and non-judgemental care. This implies that practitioners give explicit attention to individuals' circumstances. Individual therapy carries a danger of victim blaming and creating unequal power dynamics. Practitioners must therefore engage in self-reflection and avoid pathologising labels. As the causes of mental health problems appear to be multifactorial, treatment could usefully address an individual's experiences along with their existential and social needs, socio-economic struggles and challenges of maintaining their identity in an oppressive society. This requires practitioners to develop sensitivity and empathy to a wide diversity of clients, and to be aware of different groups' vulnerabilities.

2

AUSTERITY CRISIS

Psychologists for Social Change

Cheyann Heap, Christina Trigeorgis, Katherine Garzonis, Rachel Tribe, Isabella Mighetto & Joel Vos

THE PSYCHOLOGICAL IMPACT OF AUSTERITY

The term 'austerity' was initially used by politicians following the 2008 financial crash. While the UK population was subjected to austerity politics by the Conservative government, its consequences haven't been shouldered equally. People from ethnic minority backgrounds, women, LGBTQI people, people with disabilities and people with mental ill-health are all more likely to live in poverty (Joseph Rowntree Foundation, 2014). The attempt to cut the deficit by cutting welfare spending was a political choice which has elevated levels of poverty and inequality in the UK to one of the highest in the developed world (Equality Trust, 2018; United Nations, 2018). The UN Special Rapporteur on extreme poverty and human rights in the UK (2018) stated that '14 million people, a fifth of the population, live in poverty. Four million of these are more than 50% below the poverty line, and 1.5 million destitute, unable to afford basic essentials'. Following planned changes to the welfare system with universal credit, these levels are expected to rise.

In 2014, a group of likeminded people with an interest in psychology and social justice came together to form Psychologists for Social Change

(PSC), influenced by ideas from community and critical psychology. It was felt that psychologists often remained silent on political issues such as austerity, despite witnessing the psychological impact that cuts were having on individuals and communities. Now, in 2019, PSC is a national activist network, comprising connected but autonomous local groups with differing structures and emphases. PSC's members include applied psychologists, researchers, citizens, academics, therapists and students, and anyone interested in generating social and political action towards a psychologically healthier society. By synthesising existing research, members created a briefing paper outlining the impact of austerity policies on mental health (McGrath et al., 2015), identifying five 'austerity ailments': shame and humiliation; fear and distrust; instability and insecurity; isolation and loneliness; and being trapped and humiliated. Here we discuss how power, oppression and stigma intersect with some of these ailments and outline research that demonstrates how they have a long-term detrimental psychological impact on individuals and communities.

POWER AND OPPRESSION

It is important to begin with an overview of complex power relationships. 'Oppression' describes the unjust treatment of a less powerful group by a more powerful one, based on dehumanisation and denial of human rights and freedoms (Dong & Temple, 2011). Groups commonly facing oppression include women, individuals with a lower socio-economic status, black, Asian and minority ethnicity (BAME), lesbian, gay, bisexual, transgender, queer, intersex (LGBTQI) persons, and individuals with chronic or life-threatening physical disease.

People with less social power are the hardest hit by cuts to spending, services and welfare because they rely on them the most. Existing oppression, based on gender, race, ability and sexuality, is therefore exacerbated by austerity policies. Austerity driven ideals such as 'burdensomeness' (the burden to taxpayers, the burden on services, burdens of care), which often features in the social worlds of people with disabilities, create anxiety, hopelessness and worry. Burdensomeness is also a key factor in depression, psychotic experiences, bipolar disorder and suicide risk (Silva et al., 2015), and despite some suicide notes explicitly mentioning austerity and cuts they are often de-politicised (Mills, 2018). It is estimated that 80 people per month die after being found 'fit to work' (Ryan, 2015).

Women

Research indicates that women experience worse mental and physical health than men (WHO, 2000). In England, women are almost twice as likely than men to have a mental health problem (McManus et al., 2016). Research shows that women are more likely to be victims of violence and rape (UN Women, 2018); more generally, the objectification of the female body affects self-esteem (Fredrickson & Roberts, 1997). Economic discrimination also contributes to mental health; experiencing the pressure of being female in a masculine work environment, lower job positions, financial inequality and a low sense of control are all relevant issues (e.g. Lennon & Rosenfield, 1992). In addition, some women struggle with multiple roles – being a mother and working. Furthermore, women are more likely than men to be diagnosed with severe mental disorders and to be hospitalised due to gender stereotyping. Socio-cultural differences in coping may also be pertinent; research suggests that women exhibit more internalising responses (e.g. depression and anxiety) in contrast to men, who are more likely to externalise problems (e.g. with aggression and alcohol); this makes women more likely to be in contact with mental health services and men with the criminal justice system (Afifi, 2007).

Women are oppressed under austerity on a foundation of economic and social inequality, and gendered violence (Griffin, 2015). Financially, women have been disproportionately affected (Equality and Human Rights Commission, 2017), with analysis suggesting that women bear 86% of the financial burden of austerity. Women are more likely to be affected by changes such as unstable work contracts and benefits adjustments (MacLeavy, 2011). Often women are forced to choose between dependency or destitution through low wages, zero-hours contracts and unhealthy working conditions; reliance on a harsh and untenable benefits system; or insolvency (O'Brien & Kyprianou, 2017). Unequal power dynamics are thus perpetuated and reinforced by oppressive economic policies and financial structures. Austerity also echoes correlates of gendered violence, such as limited access to money and employment (Adams et al., 2008) and being closely monitored and controlled (Fletcher & Wright, 2018). It is unsurprising then that under austerity, women's mental health has worsened.

Low socio-economic status

Socio-economically disadvantaged individuals suffer disproportionately from mental health problems, but those in the middle of the social gradient are also affected (Allen et al., 2014). Individuals with lower education and poorer pay and insecure occupations experience more severe problems and suicidal thoughts (Li et al., 2011). Unemployment directly increases stress and problems such as anxiety, depression and guilt (Paul & Moser, 2009). Consequently, recessions are associated with more people suffering from common mental disorders, substance disorders and suicidal behaviour (De Almeida et al., 2018). Living in poor housing also contributes to poor mental health because of stress, uncertainty, noise from neighbours and physically unhealthy circumstances (Evans et al., 2003). The importance of good housing is underlined by research that shows how homelessness, and rough sleeping, is connected to poor physical and mental health as well as stressful experiences such as uncertainty, stigma, risk of victimisation and social isolation (Hwang, 2001).

Several explanations have been proposed to explain why adverse socio-economic circumstances lead to poor mental health. One concerns its psychological impact. Unemployment can lead to multiple forms of social exclusion: social isolation from being excluded from work; financial problems limiting participating in social events; exclusion from accessing credit or insurance facilities; and living in areas with fewer shops and cultural events (Kieselbach, 2003). Another hypothesis concerns how lack of control over one's destiny exacerbates mental health problems (Whitehead et al., 2016). Individuals need to feel efficacious and in control of their life to feel well. Although unemployment has been associated with worse mental health, there are also potential stressors at work, particularly for employees in lower-status position (Stansfeld & Candy, 2006). Their job-related stress may result from the combination of high demands and low control, while their efforts are rewarded with only a small salary. The deleterious effects of low control may be compounded by poor self-image, as toiling in low status work in an undervalued socio-economic situation can produce lower self-esteem and loss of self-efficacy (Orford, 2008). It follows that improvements to the work environment are needed, which create opportunities for autonomy, and creativity and engender trust.

Difficult political and socio-economic circumstances can make individuals prone to mental health problems, because these impact on many levels. Children raised in challenging socio-economic environments can be exposed perinatally to the poor diet, stress or lifestyle of their parents. With many stressors and fewer socio-economic opportunities to alleviate them, they are more likely to develop unhealthy lifestyles and coping behaviours. Poor diet, smoking, drinking and little physical exercise may ensue. Individuals raised in these circumstances have poorer social mobility, and as circumstances persist are more likely to experience mental health problems at later ages (Tiffin et al., 2005). Individuals with low socio-economic status are also more likely to be clustered in certain neighbourhoods that are associated with environmental complaints such as litter and graffiti, and fewer social opportunities for self-development (Pickett & Pearl, 2001).

BAME

Colonial history and ongoing neo-colonialism explicitly and implicitly influence the mental health of black, Asian and other minority ethnic groups (BAME) living in western countries. Evidence suggests that indigenous people in North America and Australia suffer from mental health problems such as depression and alcoholism, which can be traced to the historical trauma of their land being confiscated, continuing discrimination and low socio-economic status (Orford, 2008). Similarly, black people suffer from a range of mental health problems and are over-represented in prisons and mental hospitals. This can be attributed, in part, to their lower socio-economic position, although long-term intergenerational effects of oppression should also be considered.

It has been argued that their over-representation may also result from stereotyping, for example the 'angry young black man' (Fernando, 2010). Many BAME people have suffered violence and discrimination with racist incidents increasing in the last decade as alt-right, racist and fascist ideologies increase in prominence. Simultaneously, some BAME people experience stigma around mental health problems which leads them to use mental health services only for severe problems (Knifton et al., 2010). It has been argued that mental health care in western countries is insufficiently tailored to the experiences and illness perceptions of individuals with non-western backgrounds and that neo-colonial concepts exist in the therapy room (Constantine et al., 2004). Other potential sources of stress concern the cultural differences and lack of integration in the wider community (Berry & Kim, 1988). The experience of being an immigrant, of being the child or grandchild of immigrants, can lead to internal cultural conflicts, particularly when individuals have had to flee their country of origin and face the secondary trauma of seeking asylum and risking deportation (Bhugra, 2004). Negative life stories, ethnicity, social class and neighbourhood are often intertwined, again supporting a complex interactional model for the genesis of distress. Improving mental well-being then needs to incorporate improving socio-economic opportunity, fighting racism and discrimination, and improving access to community health services.

Subsequently, austerity policies specifically impact ethnic minorities in Britain in multiple ways, from housing to public mood (Thomsen, 2016). Austerity driven concepts such as scarcity, particularly with respect to resources (e.g. jobs and money), enable scapegoating which is likely to further racism-related stress (Harrell, 2000).

LGBTQI

Until 1980, the *Diagnostic and Statistical Manual of Mental Disorders* (DSM) (APA, 1980) included homosexuality as a mental disorder. Although being gay or lesbian is no longer regarded as a disorder, individuals still experience stigma and discrimination. Many gays, lesbians and bisexual individuals encounter homophobia, feel endangered or have witnessed violence against their community. Many have internalised the homophobia, which may lead to self-questioning, alcohol or drug use and mental health problems (Newcomb & Mustanski, 2010).

A group who has received specific attention for their mental health problems are transgender people – individuals who feel they are a different gender from the one assigned at birth (Erickson-Schroth & Carmel, 2016). The DSM regards 'gender dysphoria' as a mental disorder, although the World Health Organisation catalogue (WHO, 2018) does not. The diagnosis, based on limited research, has been controversial. The majority of transgender individuals experience neither mental health problems nor dysphoria, but feel their biological gender characteristics do not align with their identity (Yarbrough, 2018). Many transgender individuals experience stigmatisation and discrimination socially, but also in mental health services (Grant et al., 2010). In itself this can contribute to psychological stress.

The political context of course determines the mental health impact that being lesbian, gay, bisexual, transgender, queer or intersex (LGBTQI) has on individuals. There are 73 countries – mainly in the Middle East, Africa and Asia – where homosexual activity is illegal, and in eight countries it is punishable by death. In many of these countries an active LGBTQI subculture is tolerated as long as it is away from the public eye. However, since 2010 there has been a surge in anti-gay legislation and active policing. The International Lesbian, Gay, Bisexual, Trans and Intersex Association's (ILGA) 'State-Sponsored Homophobia Report' in 2018 describes Russia adopting a law in 2013 which has fuelled homophobia. The law forbids 'gay propaganda', effectively out lawing public expression of LGBTQI perspectives. In September 2018, Chechnya opened camps for LGBTQI people that human rights activists have branded concentration camps. Reports suggest people there are 'treated' with electric shocks, brainwashing, physical punishment and for some death. Since 2016, Indonesia has seen attacks on LGBTQI campaigners and the arrest of hundreds of consenting adults. In the US, under Trump, rights of LGBTQI people are changing, for example the banning of transgender people from military service and removing protections for transgender individuals in prisons. In general, widespread heterosexist norms have created a sense of social exclusion and stigma, leading to violence and discrimination. Consequently, LGBTQI individuals suffer disproportionately from mental health problems and suicide. Activists challenge these norms, and plea for wider acceptance of diverse sexual orientations, identities and forms of relationships.

Decreased tolerance and increased discrimination of LGBTQI individuals should be seen against the economic background. Research suggests that LGBTQI people are disproportionately affected by austerity, through work discrimination and lack of access to services (Stonewall, 2014). Despite already being underfunded, LGBTQ services have been in decline since 2009–2010, with public sector cuts and shifts in sources of funding causing problems.

Chronic & life-threatening physical illness

More than 30% of the UK population live with a chronic or life-threatening disease, a percentage which is increasing due to modern lifestyles and an aging population. Between 20% and 40% of them will experience mental health problems during their illness (Cimpean & Drake, 2011). As mental health problems lead to worse physical outcomes, lower quality of life and increased health care costs, the UK government has prioritised mental health treatment in physically ill patients (Imison et al., 2011).

National guidelines are unclear about the type of mental health support that should be provided. Currently little research is available, and traditional therapies such as cognitive behaviour therapy (CBT), cognitive stress-reduction and support groups have only modest effects (Vos, 2016). It is argued that this is because traditional therapies do not focus on patients' needs. Of course, these treatments may be helpful for some, for example those with pre-existing mental health issues. However, research on physically ill patients' needs suggest their mental health is related to their medical limitations, and specifically to how they can live a meaningful life within their physical limitations. Not surprisingly, the dominant evidence-based theories in psychology indicate that people's existential needs lie at the heart of their mental health problems. Standard treatments do not address these. Increasing numbers of mental health interventions consequently now focus on existential issues for physically ill patients. Research suggests that these recovery-oriented interventions aid mental and physical health more than traditional interventions (Vos, 2016). However, experience suggests that despite good intentions the budget for mental health care in this group is inadequate, with austerity measures only worsening an already difficult situation.

Interaction

Crucially, the above identities and related power struggles do not occur in isolation. For example, a disabled woman of colour will face a host of interacting oppressions. What we know suggests that the less social power one possesses, the more damage ensues to one's mental health (Smail, 2005). Evidence indicates that inequality, including inequality of power, is the biggest predictor of mental health problems within a society (Wilkinson & Pickett, 2009, 2018).

STIGMA

Stigma is the devaluation of a person's worth or character, based on negative perceptions of the social group to which they (apparently) belong. Stigma cannot be separated from its cultural and historical context. For example, the stigma associated with being a 'welfare queen' – a woman with children who claims out-of-work benefits – only exists in the context of political austerity (Allen et al., 2015). In a nationally representative survey, nearly half (48.7%) gave some response suggesting stigmatisation for claiming benefits (Baumberg, 2016).

Crocker and Major (1994) suggest we have less empathy for people whose stigmas are considered 'controllable'. Today, being poor or out of work is considered 'controllable', even fraudulent. This is despite the fact that 'workshy' communities do not exist (MacDonald et al., 2014), unstable working conditions are increasing, and being disadvantaged or in low-status employment is a barrier to seeking re-employment (Green et al., 2000). The consequences of such stigma include discrimination and social rejection, with corresponding low self-esteem, anxiety, depression and isolation.

Those who face welfare or poverty related prejudice may reinforce the existence of stigmatised identities in order to protect themselves psychologically from 'scroungerphobia' (Shildrick & MacDonald, 2013). Someone may use the identities of 'deserving poor' versus 'undeserving poor' to identify themselves as the part of the 'deserving' group. Baumberg (2016) found people living in high-claim areas were more likely to report internalised stigma for claiming benefits, despite it being more common within their community.

Shildrick and MacDonald (2013) suggest that cultural erosion of working-class community life, with the corresponding attrition of working-class solidarity, has made it harder to combat the stigma of poverty and claiming benefits. Therefore, individuals lacking the power of a group must resort to deflection of the stigmatised identity as they lack the power to challenge it. People are therefore required to reconstruct or disavow aspects of personal identity and group membership in order to protect themselves from the stigma that has arisen in the wake of austerity.

FEAR AND DISTRUST

Fear thrives in conditions of uncertainty and danger and abates when we feel cared for. Fear can drive people indoors, lead them to distrust others and avoid risk. When we feel ourselves or loved ones threatened, our bodies are flooded with stress hormones to prepare for an impending attack. Austerity policies that lead people to fear for their livelihoods can trigger the same reactions as a prowling tiger would have. Rates of severe anxiety and depression among the unemployed increased by more than 50% between 2012 and 2017. During this time, benefits were capped for families with children, made harder to claim and were frozen. The unemployed and those receiving welfare payments represent the most economically vulnerable, and can experience such policies as an assault on and a threat to their right to live. One study linked the recession to an additional 10,000 'economic suicides' (between 2008–2010; Reeves, 2014). Yet employment alone is no guarantee of safety. A Trades Union Congress survey in 2014 linked government cuts to heightened fears about job safety and employment security, which in turn led to increased stress, anxiety and poorer health.

Government decisions not only create fear *in* people, they can create fear *of* people. A survey by the *Independent* newspaper in 2018 (Watts, 2018) found 80% of people believed cuts to police spending had made Britain less safe. The politics of fear and the constant press coverage of the 'cash-strapped NHS' were leveraged during the Brexit campaign to argue that EU migrants put pressure on public services, despite migrants being net contributors to public finances. The British Social Attitudes survey published by the National Centre for Social Research in 2017 (Clery et al., 2017) later suggested 70% of people who voted to leave the EU were worried about immigration. Fear of our neighbours, our communities and our livelihoods encourages people to shy away from one another, impeding their ability to flourish or build resilience to certain stressors. This behaviour is passed down to our children, so although austerity is alleged to be over, its psychological effects continue. At a service and governmental level, transparency around processes and support services, especially in regard to welfare claims, can allay anxiety about what might come next and how we will cope.

HUMILIATION AND SHAME

Unlike feelings of fear and sadness, shame is a self-conscious emotion where people see themselves through the eyes of others. Shame occurs when we believe others judge us negatively and we are somehow less worthy because of who we are or what we have done. People in poverty often feel less valued by society as lower status is given to them, using words like 'guilty', 'degraded', 'useless' and 'failure' to describe how they see – or are made to see – themselves. This is reinforced through media language that humiliates: people collecting benefits are described as 'shirkers'; those in debt as 'irresponsible'; using food-banks is 'freeloading'. In areas with a large number of marginalised groups, such as immigrants, older adults and the working class, entire communities are subject to such shaming rhetoric.

Shame can be a useful emotion when it helps us correct willingly enacted behaviour. Poverty, however, is rarely a choice. Any country in recession experiences higher unemployment and job insecurity that pushes people into debt, bankruptcy and repossession. For instance, UK unemployment levels after the 2008 financial crisis rose to 8% (BBC News Online, 2015), and the proportion of households unable to meet unexpected financial expenses increased by one-third. This is not within the control of the average person, who experiences shaming messages of poverty as their responsibility while having limited means to do anything about it.

The welfare state was founded precisely because people cannot always control what happens to them and was intended to mitigate the effects of social and economic hardship. However, austerity measures have made people more vulnerable to shame and persistent poverty. This has happened in various ways: first, as seen, people accessing help are stigmatised and politicised as morally unfit – the 'undeserving poor'. This is partly because most citizens have witnessed a visible decline in public services due to austerity cuts; when people are given something for 'free' (e.g. benefit payments) and at the same time others receive less, this can be seen as unfair. Second, this decline in services and public investment removes protections people once had to reduce the impact of poverty. Freezes in public sector and social security payments mean many households are poorer, especially when combined with increased living costs. This increases distress, social exclusion and marginalisation, breaking down the trust necessary to improve education, community and work prospects, and can contribute to depression and substance misuse.

Because shame is self-conscious, it involves two sides: the self and those that 'see' you. Therefore, it cannot be improved without tackling the relationship between both sides. The first step is to prevent re-shaming, for which we already have a blueprint for services. Psychologically informed environments, where services are designed such that processes and staff reflect a better understanding of the psychological and behavioural needs of their clients, have already improved outcomes for people with mental health difficulties. A nationwide policy applying these principles to all public services, starting with welfare, would reduce re-shaming, improve overall mental health and provide more effective services to those made vulnerable by shame. Next, increasing opportunities for 'repair' in relationships empowers those with shame to help themselves.

INSTABILITY AND INSECURITY

Instability and insecurity engender uncertainty, which feeds levels of fear. However, humans cannot cope with too much fear or uncertainty, so we conduct our lives based upon mental models of what we expect will happen next. If these models are threatened (i.e. job insecurity, welfare changes or immigration reforms) potential psychological harm may ensue. Since 2012, UK workers employed in zero-hour contracts have more than tripled (from 252,000 to 901,000) (Sharma, 2018). This type of contract means that workers are not obliged to accept work offered by an employer, who is not obliged to provide contracted hours of work. This type of work, along with the booming 'gig economy', provides no long-term security. Evidence suggests that job insecurity increases levels of sickness, mental distress and worsened job performance (Broom et al., 2006). Recently, a review of longitudinal work conducted over the past 30 years concluded that job insecurity negatively influences health and well-being, specifically in relation to exhaustion, general mental/psychological well-being, self-rated health and somatic complaints (De Witte et al., 2016). Moreover, job insecurity affects the whole family. According to the Health Foundation (2018), young people could clearly see how precarious employment, along with low family income, meant that their parents were unable to support them into adulthood.

When instability and insecurity are combined with fear, isolation, stigma, inequality and oppression, segregation occurs. Segregation is the radical attempt to create security by separating 'us' from 'them'. While this brings some stability, it also isolates people from certain opportunities (affecting deprived communities most) and creates 'echo chambers'. Lacking exposure to other ways of living creates political and social polarisation without developing the empathy needed to overcome psychological barriers. This is evident in the UK today. The crux of the problem is that deprivation (be that social, economic or empathetic) breeds further deprivation. This creates groups such as the 'urban poor', a collection of disadvantaged people isolated from the mainstream economy through austerity politics. Poverty forces them into high-density, poor-quality housing, in neighbourhoods where economic and social opportunities are few and fast-food outlets are many. Interventions to increase individual health die in these environments, so poverty is compounded with ill-health. Action to help these communities cannot be done on purely an individual or local basis. Government policies focused on health inequalities or mental health distress need to address the wider social determinants, such as job insecurity.

FEELING TRAPPED AND HELPLESS

Social policy can result in people feeling trapped, powerless and helpless in different ways which, much like other austerity ailments, will be experienced differently depending on ethnicity, ability and gender. One way is through the 'poverty trap', which suggests it is harder to gain a job when you are already in poverty. When jobs are scarce, those who are already marginalised are less likely to be able to fashion a sustainable income. How difficult would this be if you have no fixed address or access to suitable clothes for an interview, transport or a mobile phone, compounded with the stress of housing and financial problems and the associated strain of being subject to stereotyping, hostility and mistrust? Cognitively, being part of this cycle teaches us that our efforts will come to naught – perhaps that we are useless, worthless or stupid. These are core thought patterns implicated in a range of mental health problems, including depression, anxiety and bipolar disorder. Indeed, failed attempts to take action to relieve stressful circumstances create learned helplessness, a key factor in the state we call 'depression'. Cuts to legal aid and community services mean people cannot find help with employment, debt, housing and other factors that may impede attempts to find work, childcare support, help for substance misuse or mental health support.

The benefits system has been likened to trauma – a critical element being, feeling trapped or helpless (Herman, 1992). Consider the mandatory five-week gap between applying for and receiving universal credit. This creates unimaginable stress for claimants who are uncertain if they can afford basic necessities. Cuts to benefit allowances and eligibility, reductions in health and social services, and the erosion of social housing can all be seen as government assaults on the right to live for the most vulnerable, resulting in real trauma. The ability to take constructive action at the time of a trauma lessens its impact (Van der Kolk, 2014). Having agency is important for recovery. On the flip side, oppressive policies and institutional structures that disempower already marginalised people, for example by being tied to insecure and low-status work for fear of unemployment, can lead to further traumatisation. Indeed, similar techniques of isolation, reducing access to money and support, and undermining self-esteem are present in the behaviours of abusive partners and the benefits system.

The long-term response to being trapped and powerless is significant. A person can become 'burnt out', physically and emotionally exhausted. For someone suffering under austerity, this may be called 'laziness', 'selfishness' or 'fecklessness'. Arguably, mental health provision under capitalism and austerity fails to acknowledge the real helplessness in someone's personal circumstances, attributing material challenges to faults within the psyche. Indeed, psychotherapy may buttress the unfair system in this way, placing responsibility onto the individual rather than the social, structural context. The system can perpetuate self-blame, where one has tried to take action and apparently 'failed'. There were 45,000 more deaths in the first four years of Conservative-led austerity policies than would have been expected if funding had remained stable (Watkins et al., 2017). As a result of austerity and cuts to services, people can become trapped in untenable home or work situations because there is no safety net to support them to escape.

ISOLATION

'There is no such thing as society.' This infamous saying of Margaret Thatcher is as apt today as it was in 1987; we are becoming a society of individuals. This is disastrous for mental health. Humans are social animals. Relating to another human is one of the first things we learn in our life, and a skill we continue refining until the day we die. Neglect is one of the most psychologically harmful forms of abuse and a threat to one's survival because it involves minimal interaction and recognition of one's basic needs. Any policy that neglects the care of its citizens or increases isolation and loneliness strikes at the heart of being human.

Isolation itself can be seen as a physical disconnection from people. Older adults in particular are more likely to spend days or weeks by themselves, which is linked to poorer well-being and delayed recovery from mental health issues. Physical health is affected too, as isolated people are at greater risk of early death (Steptoe et al., 2013). Loneliness is a psychological detachment, missing meaningful connection with others. We can be lonely even when surrounded by people, a phenomenon increasingly noticed in the digital age. Feeling that you do not mean anything to anyone, or that you have no one who means something to you, is antithetical to human existence. Loneliness is strongly linked to thoughts about suicide, which is sometimes described as a response to 'thwarted belongingness', where we looked for connection but did not find enough to make living seem meaningful. Substance misuse is also cited as an attempt to create connection, attachment and bonding when they are absent.

Despite the importance of connectedness for well-being, isolation and loneliness are characteristic features of poverty and are related to discrimination and poor access to social and community resources. Policies that reduce eligibility for welfare support, cut funding to community services or decimate affordable housing stock puts extra strain on household budgets. Less time is then spent on social activities and more on working to make ends meet. Longer working hours, further commutes and multiple jobs also reduce connection with others. Shift work in particular – which accounts for 60% of protective service workers like the police, 40% of health staff and most of the gig economy – is related to poorer mental health, physical complaints and isolation. Conversely, the higher proportion of low-paid workers in part-time work means that many families lack income to join in social activities after purchasing necessities. All of these patterns increase household stress and reduce individual and community well-being.

CONCLUSION

Considerable evidence indicates that poverty, poor housing, low income and insecure work adversely affect mental and physical health. The different 'austerity ailments' are intertwined and intersect with other forms of discrimination and disadvantage. They shape each other in ways that worsen social injustice and have ongoing, far-reaching and long-lasting psychological effects that should be recognised and considered by policy makers. The public, psychologists and frontline health care staff witness these unjust ailments on a daily basis. This witnessing must extend to taking action within health services but also in politics, to make a just and psychologically healthier society in which we all benefit.

3

THE FINANCIAL CRISIS IN MENTAL HEALTH CARE

Joel Vos

MCMENTALHEALTH

There is no such thing as a politically neutral governmental budget. All countries struggle with limited resources. Politicians therefore must decide who and what will be funded. For this they depend on civil servants, advisers and lobbyists. In this financial 'game of thrones' it is ideology that ultimately determines who wins. Budget inspections can reveal who advisers and lobbyists are and what their respective ideological positions are. It is this world behind the mental health care budget that we examine in this chapter. The crisis in this budget can be found in many countries, potentially linked to the fact that care is becoming increasingly standardised, a one-size-fits-all approach which fails many. British Secretary of State for Health and Social Care, Matt Hancock, offered a revealing insight when he said he wants the health care system to function more like McDonald's (Thompson, 2018). The McMentalHealth system that the minister envisages would see anonymous dispensers delivering 'quick fixes' but incapable of appeasing any 'mental hunger' over the long term (Binnie, 2015).

BUDGET CUTS

Worldwide, countries are spending increasing sums on mental health (WHO, 2017). However, several have seen investment stagnate because of austerity measures following the 2008 financial crisis. In the UK since then, mental health care spending has failed to increase in line with need. Child and Adolescent Mental Health Services (CAMHS) in particular are underfunded. Research points to a shortage of qualified staff and beds in mental health hospitals, with increased waiting lists (BMA, 2018). In the period 2010–2016, almost half of all mental health trusts saw budget reductions, with a 22% drop in mental health hospital beds and a 16% reduction in the number of nurses. Meanwhile, demand for services is increasing. To meet these concerns, the government earmarked funding for psychiatric research and training, and in the NHS Long Term Plan launched in January 2019 further funds for mental health were promised. However, it has been argued that more money is needed (King's Fund, 2018) for long-term investments in staff, particularly in areas previously cut (e.g. public health, social care, youth services).

ONE SIZE FITS ALL?

Since the millennium, it is apparent that many in the UK do not access mental health care, despite their need and the economic benefits of care (Layard, 2006). In response, the Labour government implemented a system to Improve Access to Psychological Therapies (IAPT). This was developed to organise and improve the delivery of, and access to, evidence-based therapies within the NHS. It is based on a 'stepped care' or triage model where 'low intensity' interventions/self-help are provided in the first instance and 'high intensity' interventions for more serious conditions. At first sight, IAPT offers interventions to suit a variety of clients. However, from its initiation, the programme has come under fire for its one-size-fits-all focus. In what follows, we will discuss why this approach is neither evidence-based nor beneficial.

One-problem-does-not-fit-all

The IAPT service has been criticised for its limited focus on specific interventions for specific clients with specific problems (anxiety and depression), ignoring individuals who fall outside this system. However, many clients present with a complex set of issues. Neither does IAPT sufficiently address comorbid mental and physical conditions.

One-treatment-does-not-fit-all

In a stepped-care model, most individuals will begin with a basic assessment and often watchful waiting (WAW) in a primary care setting. The second step involves low-intensity service (self-help, education, computerised CBT and group-based physical activity programmes). The third step comprises specific treatments for specific disorders such as depression and anxiety. The first stages usually employ cognitive-behavioural therapies, and later ones high-intensity CBT, interpersonal psychotherapy, couples therapy, brief psychodynamic therapy, counselling for depression or brief dynamic therapy. In addition to talking therapy, individuals can receive drug treatment. Individuals with more complex needs can be referred for specialised care. This model was developed with reducing cost and increasing access in mind.

The stepped-care model, despite appearances, is often more standardised. IAPT sees 900,000 people annually, with over 550,000 receiving psychological therapy and 350,000 assessment, advice and/or signposting. The majority receiving therapy get a low-intensity service or short-term standardised form of CBT. Few are referred to other therapeutic modalities. Little evidence exists that this system and these treatments are superior. Research shows that CBT is not better than humanistic counselling (Barkham & Saxon, 2018). Critical reviews also suggest that CBT trials are biased – in their design and because negative study results go unpublished. There is overwhelming evidence for the effectiveness of a range of humanistic therapies, though these have little role in IAPT (Elliott et al., 2013). There is no evidence that standardised therapies are more effective than unstandardised ones (Truijens et al., 2018). Research suggests that short-term therapies only benefit a small group of clients, whereas most require 16–20 sessions (Negt et al., 2016). Some evidence points to the cost-effectiveness and feasibility of stepped-care for depression and anxiety, but robust studies are few. In addition, research shows that stepped-care is not superior to matched care where individuals are directly allocated to a treatment that matches their needs and preferences. Thus, policy makers have created IAPT, its guidelines and pathways on the basis of a biased selection of studies with flawed designs and inconclusive findings.

One-outcome-does-not-fit-all

Performance indicators used to assess whether a service provider is successful – and thus should be paid – are mainly based on the number of clients completing treatment and the numbers who have 'recovered'. The latter is measured via routine outcome monitoring; clients routinely complete a questionnaire before the first session and after the last session. A client is deemed to have recovered if the post-treatment scores have dropped below a pre-set standard.

These questionnaires focus on testing the reduction in symptoms of depression or anxiety, the impact on work and social life, and sometimes improved scores on other disease-specific questionnaires (see Chapter 4). Thus, recovery is operationalised as scores on pre-selected questionnaires compared to a pre-set national standard. This is a narrow definition, reflecting a reductionist bureaucratic perspective. Labelling someone as 'recovered' on the basis of a single score in relation to a group norm is questionable and cannot be regarded as compelling evidence of clinically reliable change. Research shows that scores have different subjective meanings for different individuals (response bias); some dramatise their symptoms while others underestimate their impact. There is no assessment of the degree to which clients feel they have recovered in their own terms (Grey et al., 2018). Research indicates that for a majority, their needs are not directly related to symptoms measured in terms of depression, anxiety or impact on work; for them, recovery means regaining control over their life and living a meaningful and satisfying life despite their problems – which is not measured.

Economic-outcomes-do-not-fit-at-all

A key argument in the Layard Report (2006), which led to the birth of IAPT, was that it would be cost-effective and pay for itself by increasing productivity and reducing state benefits (Marks, D. F., 2018). In 2017, fewer than half of the Clinical Commissioning Groups (CCGs), who fund local mental health services, met the target (15.8%) for the number of people who should be accessing talking therapies. This means that many who needed to receive an assessment and/or treatment did not. There is also a large dropout and non-show of individuals; one of the key reasons they mention for non-attendance is the impersonality of the treatment and the rigidity of the system, particularly for ethnic minority youth (De Haan et al., 2018). Due to this lack of access and low subjective recovery rates, it is understandable that at population level, the overall prevalence of mood and anxiety disorders and symptoms has not decreased, despite increases in the provision of treatment, particularly antidepressants (Jorm et al., 2017).

In conclusion

The specific problems, treatment and outcomes of the one-size-fits-all approach does render mental health care more accessible, streamlined and standardised, like McDonald's, but it is unlikely that individual needs and experiences fit easily into this system. There is abundant evidence that a one-size-fits-all approach, whilst possibly suitable for some, fails many. Indeed, a central question for researchers is 'What works for whom?'. Instead of an approach where everyone receives the same treatment, a toolkit approach has been advocated where practitioners, after an holistic assessment of their client's needs, preferences and strengths, and in collaboration with them, employ specific tools. The focus lies on listening to the client and continuously negotiating the treatment (Cantwell et al., 2015).

MUTING VOICES

The critical voices of service users and mental health care workers are structurally mute. For instance, the most recent internal outcome report of IAPT indicates that around half the patients treated in IAPT services recover, while two-thirds show 'worthwhile benefits'. These data comes from studies coordinated by the founder of the programme, who has a clear vested interest in publishing positive results (Clark, 2018). In the first place, Clark's studies focus only on a selective subgroup with high depression scores. This is a dubious statistical ploy, as those with small depression scores can reduce their score by only a little whereas those with high scores can change much more, which can then be presented as a greater improvement; while enabling statistically significant change, such 'floor effects' do not indicate clinically reliable change. The most favourable data then is suspect and may well have been cherry picked. Furthermore, when other measures and interviews are used, only 9.2% of all adult patients experienced a recovery (Scott, 2018). Similar low rates were found for children and adolescent mental health services (Timimi, 2018). It is unsurprising that service users show different results, not only because of Clark's questionable use of data, but because research finds that routine outcome monitoring rarely correlates with the experience of service users (Lawlor et al., 2017). We would argue that, on logical grounds alone, the story of service users ought to be the most relevant.

There are several reports from service users revealing problems associated with the standardisation of care (e.g. We Need To Talk Coalition, 2017; Rethink, 2011; Beresford et al., 2010). In a large independent survey, a majority were not given a choice in their treatment, did not feel the number of sessions was sufficient, had to actively ask for support, and felt their religious-cultural needs were not considered (We Need to Talk Coalition, 2017). The 2018 independent review by the Quality Care Commission found that a majority of young people with mental health problems did not get the kind of care they needed.

It is not only the voices of service users that are ignored in the current crisis. The voices of mental health service workers also go unheard. In 2016, the Surviving Work Survey included 1,500 therapists completing questionnaires and 70 individual interviews (Cotton, 2017). The findings detailed a complex working situation, underpayment, powerlessness and fearing downgrading and deprofessionalisation of care. The atmosphere was described as high pressure due to high workload and performance management. This situation created a condition of demoralisation and depression. Participants suggested changing the management style, improving funding, better work conditions, lowering targets and improving work autonomy. They described how there were often insufficient numbers of qualified staff and supervision for the therapists, and even compared their job with a call centre due to its mechanical character. Concern was expressed about the quality of care for patients (43%) – amongst IAPT staff this increased to a staggering 58%. Many therapists raised concerns about the IAPT model, and said that they frequently did not follow its rules (Cotton, 2017).

So although researchers and managers report glowing outcomes for IAPT, service users and staff sketch a gloomy picture of NHS provision. A consistently expressed concern is of a lack of funding, a negative management style and a rigid therapeutic model. There seems to be a significant gap between the bureaucratic machine and clinical reality. The system appears ideological rather than clinical.

THE MENTAL HEALTH CARE OLIGARCHY

We have seen that governmental budgets are biased in favour of short-term therapies and psychiatric drugs despite evidence of their shortcomings. However, researchers and mental health advocates are often stonewalled by the lack of transparency regarding the mental health budget (BMA, 2018). For example, two-thirds of the budget has been officially attributed to 'other mental health workers' without further specification. One-quarter was used for psychiatrists and psychiatric nurses, whereas less than 5% was used for psychologists, social workers and occupational therapists.

The lack of transparency has not stopped several bodies from pursuing relevant data. It seems that the NHS in England spent £11.9 billion on mental health in 2017/2018, 10% of all money spent by the health department (FullFact, Mental Health, 2018). Most of this goes to CCGs (groups of GPs and other doctors who buy health services in their region); the remainder goes to specialist/secondary care services provided by hospitals/trusts. The Children's Commissioner (2017) found that around 6% of the budget is used for children and young people, a figure below the proportion of the population they comprise. Evidence indicates that less funding is allocated to talking therapies than other treatments. Furthermore, many CCGs and trusts have increased their budgets for IAPT, while decreasing their budget for secondary care and other treatments (BMA, 2018). One of the few increases in expenses are psychiatric drugs, with 80 million annual prescriptions in the UK and a budget of half a billion pounds (NHS, 2017). In summary, information shows that the biggest winners in the budget allocation are managers, trainers, psychiatrists, IAPT services and psychopharmaceutical companies; the biggest losers are secondary care, humanistic/relational therapies, and talking therapies in general.

Who then are the decision makers and how are decisions made about the mental health care budget? The initial lobbyists for IAPT comprised mostly cognitivists, psychiatrists and behaviourists with clear personal interests in promoting CBT. Many of the positive research findings for IAPT come from members of this lobby group. Our inspection of the CVs of the contributors to the clinical guidelines and pathways show that 83% have connections with CBT or the psychopharmaceutical industry (www.nice.org.uk/, obtained in November 2018). All told, this suggests that unhealthy vested interests may be operating. So when IAPT was launched on World Mental Health Day in 2007, it was not surprising that only CBT was provided as standard mental health care.

Several authors have accused IAPT of being overly focused on CBT (Timimi, 2015a, 2015b) and that where other approaches are included, they lack proportional attention to relational and humanistic therapies, and remain dependent on inadequate diagnostic categories. Although IAPT has slightly opened its doors to non-CBT approaches, the politics and funding remain focused on CBT, brief therapies and psychopharmaceutical drugs.

Treatments included in IAPT need first to be approved by the National Institute for Health and Care Excellence (NICE), an 'independent organisation responsible for providing evidence-based guidance on health and social care'. NICE's charter states that it looks at both clinical outcomes and cost-effectiveness. Its guidelines mention a wide collection of sources of clinical evidence, but the focus is on systematic literature reviews and meta-analyses of quantitative studies. Quantitative studies use measurement instruments that have been selected on the basis of theoretical expectations of possible treatment outcomes. This means that if a patient in a trial has experiences about the treatment which do not fit the pre-determined outcome categories, this will not be reported. As IAPT focuses on the reduction of depression and anxiety, the guidelines have been developed on the basis of providing quantitative evidence for this.

The main focus of NICE lies in cost-effectiveness. Specifically, how much an intervention improves quality of life and how much it costs. Most quality-of-life instruments that are used in the cost-effectiveness studies cited in the NICE guidelines focus on physical symptoms and practical issues and less on recovery measures that clients prioritise as therapy outcomes. Furthermore, the focus on anxiety and depression as clinical outcomes creates a bias towards interventions that could temporarily improve these symptoms without changing the client's fundamental well-being over the long-term.

Quantitative research indicates that humanistic and relational therapies have large effects on improving self-efficacy, meaning in life, hope and social relationships (Vos, 2018; Elliott et al., 2013). Such quantitative and qualitative outcomes are more in line with the needs and preferences of clients than the quality of life indices used in cost-effectiveness instruments. As mentioned above, research indicates that there is little or no correlation between such quantitative outcomes and the subjective experiences of clients when they are asked to speak openly outside of the pre-selected outcome categories. Clients are not asked about their subjective needs and preferences before they start therapy, nor the extent to which these are satisfied by the health service (Grey at al., 2018), nor their views of the process of therapy. Standard clinical outcome measures do not show the extent to which clients feel the treatment helps them to live a meaningful and satisfying life. Consequently, service users' experiences are structurally neglected in research, guidelines and budget allocation.

DISCUSSION

This chapter has shown how mental health care suffers under budget cuts and McDonaldisation. A standardised approach prevails that, despite lacking empirical support, is promoted by a small powerful group with direct interests to mould the system in their favour. What is the bigger organisational picture behind the resultant financial crisis? Why is mental health care reduced to pharmaceutical and cognitive-behavioural interventions delivered in short semi-standardised sessions? In later chapters, we will discuss some possible answers.

4

BIOMEDICAL AND DRUG CRISIS

James Davies

Over the last 10 years criticism of psychiatric diagnosis has grown in both volume and credibility. In regard to the controversy surrounding the 2013 publication of DSM-5, in that year alone over 100 critical editorials, op-eds and articles were published in the press, alongside an array of articles in academic journals (Ledford, 2013; Bracken et al., 2012). These charged DSM-5 with over-medicalising human suffering by lowering diagnostic thresholds and expanding the number of 'mental disorders' with which people can be diagnosed. Such criticisms gained unprecedented professional support in late 2012, when over 50 mental health organisations internationally (including British Psychological Society, American Psychoanalytic Association, Danish Psychological Society and American Counselling Association) signed an online petition calling for a halt to the publication of DSM-5. During that same period many critical books drew public attention to the problems of psychiatric diagnosis more broadly (e.g. Frances, 2013; Davies, 2013). These works highlighted the unscientific manner in which diagnostic manuals and tools are contrived and deployed, the poor reliability and validity of psychiatric diagnosis, the conflicts of interests between DSM committees and the pharmaceutical industry, and the stigma psychiatric labels invariably induce.

In 2019 the critical momentum has not abated, with books, articles and public debate continuing to flood public and professional discourse, and new organisations and movements being inaugurated by international cohorts of mental health professionals (e.g. Global Summit on Diagnostic Alternatives, Drop the Disorder initiative, Power Threat Meaning Framework and Hearing Voices Network). These initiatives are actively developing, evaluating, advocating and disseminating alternatives to current diagnostic thinking. In short, the burgeoning international criticism of the making and assigning of psychiatric labels is no longer confined to a small subset of intellectuals and survivors previously dismissed as 'anti-psychiatrists', but now constitutes a mainstream and authoritative social movement, such is the conviction in large sections of the mental health, media, survivor and service-user communities that the medical model of distress is failing those in need.

The purpose of this chapter, then, will be to revisit some of these critical arguments in addition to articulating new ones. In particular, I shall focus on what Robert Whitaker (2017) referred to as the 'economies of influence' – those conflicts of interests that have aided diagnostic expansion, and thus the over-medicalisation and medicating of our behavioural and mental states. In short, if we are to move beyond the current biomedical paradigm of emotional distress to embrace more effective non-medical alternatives, then identifying the failings of our current approach is a necessary step.

THE CONSTRUCTION OF DIAGNOSTIC MANUALS

Diagnostic manuals such as the DSM and the International Classification of Diseases (ICD) have expanded the number of mental disorders over consecutive editions. In the last 50 years the DSM has more than tripled the number of mental disorders believed to exist, from 106 in the 1960s to approximately 370 today. In addition, the diagnostic thresholds people must meet to receive a diagnosis have been progressively lowered (Frances, 2013), resulting in more types of suffering being captured by diagnostic criteria than at any time in the past. Taken together, these processes have led to what has been called 'diagnostic inflation' or 'over-medicalisation' – phrases denoting the unjustified reclassification of many natural and normal (albeit painful) human responses to the problems of living as 'mental disorders' requiring medical intervention.

Diagnostic inflation did not emerge from any advances in biological research (there are still no discovered bio-markers for most 'mental disorders'), but from the consensus-based and culturally situated judgments of small and purposely selective groups of DSM and ICD committee members. Research has exposed the arbitrary and culture-bound processes by which diagnostic systems were contrived and expanded by such committees (Davies, 2013). In the absence of any guiding neurobiological research, and in the face of contradictory and incomplete clinical data, small diagnostic committees throughout the history of psychiatry have relied on reaching consensus among themselves about how disorders should be defined, where to set diagnostic thresholds and whether or not to add or remove diagnoses. Archival and oral histories of how such consensus was formed, at least during the construction of DSM, have paid careful attention to the processes leading to committee consensus. This research has shown that committee voting was a central mechanism by which key DSM conclusions were decided regarding how to define disorders, whether or not to include them, and where to set thresholds for receiving them (Davies, 2017).

While it goes without saying that voting is not a scientific activity, some may argue that the more recent editions of ICD and DSM were based on more scientifically robust activities. While this argument has been advanced, there remains no evidence to substantiate it. One reason for this is that the processes governing the construction of later manuals (e.g. DSM-5) remain opaque. For example, members of the DSM-5 taskforce were asked to sign confidentially agreements by the publishers, the APA, prohibiting them from discussing DSM's construction after the fact; furthermore, the APA has embargoed all materials pertaining to DSM-5's construction till 15 years post publication, making any objective assessment of DSM's construction impossible to undertake. Additionally, even if the argument could be made that later processes were robust, it is noteworthy that the construction of DSM is a cumulative process (each edition building upon the last). Therefore, most inclusions ratified by vote in the 1980s live on through DSM-5 today.

THE PSYCHIATRIC DRUG CRISIS AND EPIDEMIC

While it is therefore right to discount DSM and ICD as credible scientific works (they are works of *psychiatric culture*, not of science), we can take the critique further by showing how these cultural artefacts have inflicted harm – not only by stigmatising the human propensity to suffer (suffering is no longer a natural and understandable human protest, but a biomedical disorder of the self) but also since the over-medicalisation caused by diagnostic inflation has driven increases in psychiatric prescribing since the 1990s (Kleinman, 2012; Paris, 2013).

So successful has the medicalisation/medicating regime been that in many industrialised nations today over 20% of the adult population was prescribed a psychiatric medication last year alone (2017–18).

To understand this figure, and focusing on antidepressants alone, over 7.3 million people were prescribed antidepressants in England in 2016–17 (DHSC, 2018) – 16% of the entire English adult population – with the number of individual annual prescriptions now topping 65 million (NHS Digital, 2017). Not only are prescribing rates increasing, so too is the average length of time people spend on the drugs, which has doubled since the mid-2000s in the UK.

Why antidepressants are being taken for longer periods can be partly explained in the light of evidence revealing that our current guidelines on antidepressant withdrawal (NICE, 2009; APA, 2010) significantly underestimate the commonality, severity and duration of the adverse withdrawal symptoms people experience when trying to stop the drugs – an underestimation potentially leading to withdrawal reactions being misdiagnosed, as relapse, with drugs being reinstated as a consequence (Davies & Read, 2018). This state of affairs is both upsetting and bemusing as it suggests that many people are becoming trapped on drugs that are, for most people, no more effective than placebos and which only show minor (clinically insignificant) improvements over placebo for the most severely distressed (Cipriani et al., 2018). In short, while for most people the differences between placebo and antidepressant are clinically insignificant, unlike placebo, antidepressants elicit side-effects for between 40–70% of people taking them as well as withdrawal effects for around 50%, effects that, by being misdiagnosis or not tolerated, fuel longer durations of use.

Rising long-term antidepressant use is of concern. In addition to the obvious economic costs incurred, the human costs are serious, as long-term use is associated with increased severe side-effects, impaired autonomy and resilience, weight gain, worsening outcomes for some people, poorer long-term outcomes for depression, greater relapse rates and increased risk of neurodegenerative disease (Kendrick, 2015; Hengartner et al., 2018; Maslej et al., 2017; Davies & Read, 2018). With antipsychotics the situation is similar; long-term use is associated with increased risks of serious adverse cardiovascular, metabolic and neurological side effects (Salvo et al., 2016), decreased social functioning and worsening symptomatology (Harrow et al., 2012).

Research showing the harms of long-term use is crucial when realising that wherever we see longer and more widespread use, mental health disability claims increase. Over the last 20 years rates of mental health disability in the UK have doubled, with similar increases seen across the developed world (Whitaker 2016). The fact that we can observe this correlation across different countries (all with dissimilar health systems, levels of inequality etc.) obliges us to consider the extent to which the adverse effects of the drugs – particularly antidepressants – are fuelling the global burden of mental health disability. Given the importance of these considerations as well as the harmful effects that psychiatric drug can elicit, it is vital to assess both how drug consumption is being fuelled by medicalisation and its aggressive industrial promotion.

INDUSTRY INFLUENCE ON MEDICALISATION

How then does the relationship between medicalisation and rising psychiatric drug consumption operate? What mechanisms of influence does industry exert to expand drug consumption via medicalisation? In order to address this question directly, it will be useful to distinguish between *direct* and *indirect* forms of industry influence.

In the first case, *direct* influence denotes the undertaking of activities explicitly designed to increase prescribing, such as direct marketing and advertising initiatives. As this type of influence is clear in form and intent, and as its effects have been extensively covered elsewhere (Greenslit, 2005), I shall restrict myself to focusing on *indirect* industry influence. This latter process broadly denotes a form of financial influence harder to spot, one invariably operating by proxy and/or purposeful default; that is, via the financial sponsoring of persons, institutions or apparatuses deemed sympathetic and/or potentially advantageous to the expansion of psychopharmaceutical markets.

An obvious example of indirect influence occurs through industry financially sponsoring 'key opinion leaders' in the mental health and psychiatric field. When researchers at the University of Massachusetts inspected the financial interests of those who sat on the various committees of DSM-IV, they exposed the extent to which this kind of influence operates. Of the 170 people constructing DSM-IV, a full 95 (56%) had one or more financial associations with the pharmaceutical industry; and on those committees that oversaw the 'disorders' for which drugs are the first-line treatment, 88% had drug company financial ties (Cosgrove et al., 2006).

This form of indirect influence is so powerful due to how typical and routine it has become within the psychiatric profession; a normalisation that has inoculated many to the true depth of their biasing effects. This normalisation was illustrated to me at a debate in the Houses of Parliament in June 2013, when I raised the issue of industry payments with the Chair of DSM-IV, Allen Frances. He responded that while the DSM committee essentially comprised 'good guys' who wanted to do a good job, maybe it was remiss that DSM-IV lacked a conflict of interest policy at the time it was developed, explaining that in the 1990s such financial ties were not deemed relevant enough to warrant declaration.

While DSM-IV had no conflict of interest policy, DSM-5 (APA, 2013) certainly did. This was partly owing to other areas of medicine, during the mid-2000s, exposing the biasing effects such conflicts generate and advocating for transparency. Following this trend, broader transparency was introduced to DSM-5. The result was that of the 29 people charged with writing the manual, 21 were revealed as having previously received honoraria, consultancy fees or funding from pharmaceutical companies, including the Chair of the Task Force, David Kupfer, and the Vice Chair, Darrel Regier (Davies, 2013).

While those possessing financial ties often dismiss or downplay their biasing effects, research suggests that they prejudice recipients towards favouring psychopharmaceuticals in their clinical, educational and research activities (Orlowski & Wateska, 1992; Lexchin et al., 2003). Given DSM has medicalised swathes of painful normality, driving up drug prescriptions as a consequence, it is concerning that those responsible for over-medicalisation were financially linked to the companies set to benefit from the expansion of drug consumption that over-medicalisation has engineered (Davies, 2017).

My second example of indirect influence relates to diagnostic practices within the NHS, and in particular to two of the most influential mental health diagnostic tools administered in UK: the patient questionnaires, PHQ-9 and GAD-7. From the mid-2000s these documents began being used throughout primary care to enable GPs to assess whether a person has depression (PHQ-9) or anxiety (GAD-7), and if so, how severely.

A major criticism of both is that they set a low bar for what constitutes having a form of depression or anxiety for which medication should be prescribed. For instance, if you indicate on PHQ-9 that in the 'last two weeks' you have 'nearly every day' experienced poor appetite, troubled sleep, low concentration and energy, you qualify for the diagnosis of 'moderate depression', which, according to NHS guidelines, is sufficient grounds for prescribing an antidepressant. That PHQ-9 has such a low bar becomes more concerning when we discover that these instruments were developed by, their NHS distribution paid for by, and their copyright owned by Pfizer Pharmaceuticals – a company that makes two of the most prescribed anti-anxiety and antidepressant drugs in the UK: Effexor (venlafaxine) and Zoloft (sertraline). In short, allowing a pharmaceutical company to set clinical thresholds for what constitutes having a form of depression or anxiety for which their drugs should be prescribed is an example of how indirect industry influence works.

My final example of *indirect* influence draws upon a personal anecdote. During a research trip to New York City in November 2013, a colleague drew my attention to the fact that the number one best-selling book in the US at that time was DSM-5, and that it had been within the top 10 for six months since its publication. To get a sense of scale, a very popular book at the time, *Harry Potter*, was languishing at number five, while *Fifty Shades of Grey*, recently published, floundered at number eight. Additionally, DSM-5 was hardly cheap, with the paperback version costing $88. So why were so many people buying DSM-5?

I raised this question the following day in a meeting with a psychology professor at New York University. Given her work in primary care in the New York State area, she had discovered the reason that DSM sales were so high was because the pharmaceutical industry had been buying the DSM in bulk and distributing it freely to clinicians up and down the state. In her view, why the industry would do this was obvious: 'As almost any kind of suffering is caught by the DSM, disseminating DSM is just good business: it drives up diagnosis rates and ... prescriptions.'

While the above illustration remains to be definitively verified, it is consistent with other indirect methods by which industry has promoted psychiatric drugs historically, especially with respect to their targeting academic and clinical professionals in order to drive up prescription rates. Since the 1990s, the pharmaceutical industry has been a major financial sponsor of UK and US academic psychiatry, significantly influencing research, training and practice (Gøtzsche, 2013). This influence has been exerted through many heads of psychiatry departments receiving departmental income from drug companies, while at the same time receiving personal income (Campbell et al., 2007); through nearly all clinical trials into psychiatric drugs being pharmaceutically financed; through most academic drug researchers receiving research funding, consultancy fees, speakers fees or other honoraria from industry; and through leading psychiatric organisations, such as the American Psychiatric Association (the publisher of DSM), receiving most of its operational costs from industry (e.g. with such support the APA's annual revenues rose from $10.5 million in 1980, to $50.2 million by 2000; Whitaker, 2017).

That pharmaceutical companies have actively used their extensive financial power to shape practice and ideology within the mental health field, driving up prescription rates, is no surprise. But the extent to which such companies have promoted over-medicalisation (i.e. have concertedly targeted how we think about human distress in order to normalise prescribing) is not fully appreciated. Anthropologists, in particular, have shown in detail how pharmaceutical companies have purposively translated local, non-medical languages of distress into western, medicalised, DSM-based nomenclature in order to create new markets for pharmaceutical products (Skultans, 2003; Ecks, 2005). The anthropologist, Stefan Ecks (2005), termed this process 'metaphysical globalisation', where the dissemination of DSM and ICD classifications in new locales becomes an essential step in expanding psycho-pharmaceuticals into new markets.

Anthropologists like Skultans have analysed such processes of 'metaphysical globalisation' at play. Examining Latvia, she showed that following the translation of ICD into Latvian, pharmaceutical companies funded large campaigns to 'educate' Latvian psychiatrists and family doctors about the new diagnostic category of depression. This led to the gradual reconceptualisation of one local understanding of distress – *nervi* – into the western category of 'clinical depression'. The concomitant shift in practice (from investigating the possible social and political meanings of *nervi*, to treating 'depression' pharmacologically) led to *nervi* being depoliticised and reconfigured as a medical problem, which opened up a brand-new market for antidepressant drugs.

Similar mechanisms were analysed in Japan (Kitanaka, 2013) during GlaxoSmithKline's (GSK) marketing of its antidepressant, Seroxat, in the early 2000s. At that time the Japanese category closest to depression, *utsybyo*, described a chronic illness as severe as schizophrenia and for which suffers needed hospitalisation. Therefore, large swathes of the less severely distressed, who get prescribed selective serotonin reuptake inhibitors (SSRIs) in Europe and the US, resided outside the pool of consumers companies could target. As a result, GSK undertook a campaign to convince these untreated people to think of their diverse forms of moderate distress as 'depression' and as treatable with Seroxat. While TV adverts were funded to market the condition, approximately 1,350 Seroxat-promoting medical representatives visited selected doctors an average of twice weekly, priming them to prescribe Seroxat to the coming influx of 'depressed' patients (Schulz, 2004). Depression websites and web communities were also established by GSK, being made to look like grassroots movements. As a result, the category of depression gained wide cultural salience, and Seroxat sales rose to $200 million in the two years following the campaign (Davies, 2013).

While I offer only two examples above, similar processes have been observed by anthropologists in many countries, prompting some to argue that the global spread of psychiatric disease classifications and diagnostic routines can help account for the vast global increases in antidepressant use (Ecks, 2005). Pharmaceutical companies would likely contend that these promotional activities – at home and abroad – are justified on the grounds that they advanced health care to those who would otherwise be denied effective treatments. By educating populations into the virtues of the medical management of emotional/social/psychological distress, their promotional activities perform a vital public and human service.

Of course, where psycho-technologies genuinely help the distressed, these arguments have some currency. However, research has shown that the safety and efficacy of psychiatric drugs has been exaggerated by both industry and those professionals whom industry funds, and that growing consumption of such drugs has been driven less by clinical success than by good marketing concealing bad science (Greenslit, 2005), the manipulation and burying of negative clinical trials data (Kondro & Sibbald, 2004), lax medicines regulation (Healy, 2006), poor provision for non-drug alternatives (UKCP, 2015), and strong financial allegiances between industry and psychiatry (Campbell et al., 2007; Cosgrove et al., 2006). In short, the argument that pharmaceutical promotion has placed sufferers needs before its shareholders' is difficult to substantiate.

CONCLUSION

In this chapter I have outlined certain dynamics linking industry influence, the over-medicalisation of suffering and the over-prescribing of psycho-pharmaceuticals. If I were to trace a causal chain of events, the first factor – industry influence – enables all that follows, which, from the standpoint of industry, is the point: such influence is a costly investment from which a return is expected (one that can only result from increasing diagnoses and prescriptions). While industry influences drive medicalisation and over-prescribing, it would be remiss to ignore that industry itself is only capable of wielding such influence because of the weak legislative checks and balances upon its activities. In short, wider sociological analyses as to what enables such carte blanche influence are essential in understanding why over 20% of our adult population was prescribed a psychiatric medication last year alone. To understand the drivers of this epidemic we must move beyond assessing the interests and practices of psychiatry and industry (important as they are), to inspecting the systemic political/economic arrangements in which such interests are allowed to thrive, despite worsening clinical outcomes and growing evidence of drug harms. In short, the current biomedical crisis is not just to do with over-medicalisation and over-prescribing, and the evident harms of each, but the factors permitting these processes to operate unchecked.

5

DIAGNOSTIC CRISIS

James Davies

In the previous chapter I examined links between industry, over-medicalisation and over-prescribing. The implication was that the latter two processes are outcomes of the extent to which industry has been permitted to exert unprecedented influence over how we, as a society, have come to understand, manage and respond to emotional distress. In this chapter I wish to focus more closely on the idea that the diagnostic process itself – championed, funded and promoted by industry, and essential to the performance of widespread prescribing – is good for the people it targets. I will challenge this view by highlighting ways in which traditional diagnostic processes harm those they purport to help. While this standpoint remains controversial, we should not underestimate its growing credibility and appeal for increasing numbers of mental health professionals who are only too aware, through their own professional practice, of the mixed blessings psychiatric labels afford. Given the mounting appetite for non-diagnostic alternatives, it is important to spell out some major criticisms of diagnosis in mental health. In what follows I shall provide six reasons why the value and utility of psychiatric diagnosis must be contested.

PSYCHIATRIC DIAGNOSIS IS NORMATIVE

The impulse to classify diverse phenomena (whether biological, material or social) is both fundamentally human and, as anthropologists have shown, universal. What is interesting about diagnostic systems, however, is that they do not merely classify different kinds of suffering. They take the further step of pronouncing upon the meaning of that suffering. There is nothing normative about classifying birds into big and small, until I introduce the cultural prejudice that big birds are better. And that is precisely where our classificatory systems transgress mere description: they are medically loaded meaning systems, which implicitly pathologise the phenomena they slice and dice. Our classificatory systems, while posing as disinterested works of phenomenology, are actually highly invested, value-laden (and experience-shaping) works of cultural description.

Diagnostic systems, then, bring to the different species of suffering they classify the medical and pathologising philosophy they claim to derive from them. In this sense they assume what they should rather demonstrate: that the suffering they categorise is in fact medical 'illness', 'disorder' or 'dysfunction' rather than the organism's call for some kind of necessary change; or our understandable reaction to hurt, trauma or impairment; or an instance of what anthropologists have termed 'social suffering' – namely, a non-pathological, distressing, yet comprehensible human response to harmful social, political, relational and environmental conditions (Kleinman, 1997; Kitanaka, 2013). Put differently, framing emotional distress in medical terms betrays a particular philosophical preference, one detached from any biological foundation. It betrays a situated and subjective interpretation of facts – one still entirely hypothetical. It is in this sense that Sedgewick (1982: 30) was correct when stating that 'the natural events of suffering do not constitute diseases, illness or pathology prior to the human social reasons we attach to them'. Rather they only *become* such medical 'facts' when seen through a culturally situated medical lens.

The recasting of suffering as medical 'illness' (while highly profitable to industry and a brand of psychiatric ideology) forecloses the idea that suffering can have any purposive value. This establishes problems for professionals who seek to galvanise recovery in others by encouraging their expectation that such recovery will occur. One common struggle for mental health professionals is inviting clients to consider the potential meanings of their distress (beyond its being simple biological affliction). This is difficult if the client has already succumbed to a biomedical view of their predicament: that their suffering is a biological 'illness' that may well be chronic. Accordingly, all that can be hoped for is a more or less successful management of 'symptoms' or, if 'symptoms' abate, a lengthy period of 'remission'. To illustrate briefly how such beliefs can work on sufferers, I offer the following vignette of a young man I interviewed during placement in a psychiatric day centre.

> Two months before I met Peter, he had been sectioned under the Mental Health Act 1983 for a failed suicide attempt. Peter told me his psychiatrist had subsequently diagnosed him with schizoaffective disorder for which a daily dose of clozapine was prescribed. When I asked him how he expected things to turn out, he told me that his psychiatrist had said that his condition was incurable, hence the importance of continuing – perhaps indefinitely – to take his medication. As I spoke further to Peter, it was clear that the idea he may have a life-long 'condition' filled him with hopelessness and dread that his 'condition' would worsen. Identifying as mentally ill now made him deeply anxious about his future.

As the work of the anthropologist Emily Martin (2009) has shown, fatalism or fears of deterioration commonly arise in those diagnosed with a severe 'mental disorder'. While a diagnosis may initially be experienced as validating, creating the illusion that you are understood (and so will be helped), it can also stoke anxiety about non-recovery or deterioration. Being diagnosed, therefore, can heighten the fear of never getting better or else 'going mad', which can in turn foster dependency upon those socially positioned as experts. In such events it is harder for people who have developed such dependency to attribute the cause of any actual deterioration to those upon whom they've come to depend, or upon the medical narrative and 'treatments' in which they have placed their hopes. If the 'condition' worsens, it is the 'condition' itself that must be blamed, not the system of ideas, nor the 'treatment' by which the 'condition' has been framed.

While in psychiatry there is a ritual of label ascription, there is rarely one of label removal. The latter belies the notion that severe 'mental illness' can only be managed, never cured. Such messages about the 'chronicity' of mental illnesses, despite their contested validity and utility (Timimi, 2013), often breed counter-productive fatalism, varying degrees of hopelessness, fear of deterioration and continued dependence upon the system maintaining that fatalism. These are all factors that undermine recovery by threatening the 'expectation of recovery' so important to working productively through one's distress. As the work of Meyer et al. (2002) made clear, people who expect to get better as a result of their 'treatment' have better outcomes than those who don't. Anything undermining such expectations, especially when cloaked as essential treatment, mitigates the good outcomes they were designed to achieve.

While the above has referred to a shift towards fatalism that can often follow being diagnosed, interestingly, a similar shift has also been observed in medical students as they undergo residency training in psychiatry. It was found that before undergoing their psychiatric rotation, general medical students 'did not endorse stereotypes commonly attached to [people with schizophrenia], such as being dangerous, lazy or of lower intelligence'. By the end of their psychiatry rotation, however, 'more students were found to believe that [people with schizophrenia], cannot recover, have no insight into their condition, cannot make reasonable decisions, cannot work in regular jobs and are dangerous to the public' (Economou et al., 2012). While it is difficult to extrapolate from this study to all medical students, it nevertheless shows that negative fatalism about human suffering can be *instilled*, either by way of the persuasions of professional training or by way of the authoritative declarations made in 'clinical care'.

PSYCHIATRIC DIAGNOSIS IS NOT RELIABLE

It has long been recognised that there are no known biological or physical tests that can verify any psychiatric diagnosis (Bentall, 2012). This is because for all 'mental disorders', except dementia and some rare chromosomal conditions, no biological markers have been identified. The absence of such tests therefore renders psychiatric diagnosis highly unreliable. The full extent of this problem was first recognised in the early 1970s (e.g. Cooper et al., 1972), when tests were designed to measure 'diagnostic reliability' (i.e. the degree of likelihood that two separate psychiatrists would independently assign a patient the same label).

Such trials revealed that for many 'disorders' two psychiatrists in the same location would assign different diagnoses to the same patient between 32–42% of the time (Carlat, 2010), a figure which has hardly improved for many diagnoses over the subsequent 40 years (Aboraya et al., 2006). For instance, the most recent field trials for DSM-5 (2013) have shown that for categories like 'major depressive disorder', 'generalised anxiety disorder', 'obsessive compulsive disorder' and 'schizoaffective disorder', two psychiatrists will reach disagreement over the diagnosis around 30–40% of the time, and for diagnoses like 'bi-polar II' and 'schizophrenia' between 15–20% of the time (Freedman et al., 2013). These results become more concerning when we realise that they were obtained in highly controlled academic settings, where the interviewers were very prepared, the patients carefully selected, and where there was no time pressure to issue a diagnosis. In the real, more chaotic, time-strapped world of practice, we can expect lower reliability rates (Frances, 2012).

Other factors attesting to low reliability of psychiatric diagnosis are the frequency with which people are diagnosed with more than one condition – co-morbidity – (Timimi, 2013), and the frequency with which a person's main diagnosis is changed. To illustrate the detrimental impact of this latter practice, consider the following vignette, which concerns a middle-aged woman I came to know, once again, during a psychiatric observation placement.

> In 1997, Sarah, as I shall call her, had been diagnosed with 'bi-polar disorder'. Over the following seven years she was admitted into hospital as an inpatient many times. A week before meeting Sarah her diagnosis unexpectedly changed. Her new consultant psychiatrist disagreed she suffered from bi-polar disorder, informing her that 'borderline personality disorder' seemed 'a better fit'. As I came to know Sarah a little more over subsequent weeks, it emerged that this event had thrown her into a period of deep instability. Her bi-polar diagnosis had for many years not only determined the drugs she had been prescribed, but also the identity she had assumed. If she agreed with her new consultant her identity would have to change, but if she disagreed she would be defying the very medical authority whose infallibility she had come to crave.

I wondered whether her questions would lead her to greater confusion, self-doubt and finally towards deeper dependence upon the very system she doubted, or else to the birth of more questioning, less deference, more self-reliance and finally to an emerging willingness to explore non-medical ways of understanding and managing her distress.

While I never discovered the outcome of Sarah's predicament, her story illustrates that poor diagnostic reliability is not just a technical problem but a fundamentally human problem for those being misdiagnosed, unnecessarily diagnosed or subjected to diagnostic change. Psychiatric diagnoses are not, after all, impotent categories, but vigorously resonant cultural symbols that have powerful implications for those over whom they come to preside.

THE STIGMA AND SELF-STIGMA OF DIAGNOSIS

The stigma and self-stigma can that invariably follow receiving a psychiatric diagnosis is one of the most publicised adverse effects of psychiatric intervention, one recognised by supporters and critics of diagnosis alike. Stigma can adversely affect recipients' employment prospects; it can undermine their relationships, social standing and self-respect. People labelled with 'depression' are more likely to be viewed as having character flaws, being personally weak, lazy and unpredictable

(Hinshaw, 2007). Such negative perceptions have become so entrenched that an estimated 92% of people in Britain believe that admitting to having a 'mental illness' would harm their career (Time to Change, 2015). Such beliefs appear justified. A study in *The Lancet* involving around 1,000 depressed people in 35 countries found that 79% of those diagnosed reported experiencing discrimination (Lasalvia et al., 2013).

The deleterious effects of stigma not only stem from the negative reactions of others, but also from the subtler insidious effects of adopting the 'sick role', otherwise known as 'self-stigma'. Consider the case of Eleanor Longden, a psychiatric patient turned professional psychologist.

> As a young psychology student Eleanor began hearing voices during her first term at university. Like many people of her age she harboured insecurities, but what marked her out was the voice she heard, which began to narrate many things she did. Although in its early days the voice was 'neutral, unthreatening ... and reassuring', she noticed that on occasion, 'it's calm exterior sometimes slipped, it occasionally mirrored my own unexpressed emotion ... if I was angry and had to hide it ... then the voice would sound frustrated' (Longden, 2013). Events took a dramatic turn when she told a friend about the voice. Her friend's subsequent fear that she should seek medical help was infectious, and suddenly the voice no longer seemed so benign. Things degenerated further after a psychiatric assessment, which led to a diagnosis of schizophrenia and to hospitalisation. Now believing her voice was an index of psychiatric sickness, her relationship to it became hostile. As she recalled, 'this represented taking an aggressive stance towards my own mind, engaging in "a kind of psychic civil war"' (ibid.). Proportionate to her growing mistrust the voice became more menacing. Soon after her diagnosis she experienced a toxic, tormenting sense of hopelessness, humiliation and despair, about herself and her prospects (ibid.). Two years later the voices had become so bad that she tried to remove them by drilling a hole in her head.

It is important to note that Eleanor's voices took a sinister turn only once she began to interpret them as symptoms of pathology. This recasting of experience into pathological terms worsened her state, as now there was annexed to the original experience the additional fear, confusion and shame of believing herself to be chronically mentally ill. It is also important to note the timing of Eleanor's improvement, which occurred only after she began to engage with others – fellow survivors, fellow voice hearers, a compassionate doctor – who taught her to view her voices differently. From these she learned an alternative version of events: her voices were not an index of pathology but 'a meaningful response to traumatic life events, particularly to childhood events … [and] as such [they] were not my enemies but a source of insight into solvable emotional problems' (Longden, 2013). Once she began to read her voices metaphorically rather than literally – exposing her fears – her management of them altered. She learnt to set boundaries for the voices and interact with them assertively yet respectfully. In time, she learnt to collaborate with them by interpreting them as closely related to aspects of herself that carried, as she put it, 'overwhelming emotions that I'd never had an opportunity to process or resolve; memories of sexual trauma and abuse, of anger guilt shame low self worth' (ibid.). It was by means of this alternative model of understanding and managing her voices that Eleanor gradually renounced the medical view of her predicament, withdrew from her medication, and overcame her despair.

The case of Eleanor's is indicative of many people who have adopted a similar interpretative stance to voice hearing and to demonstrably useful effect (Longden et al., 2017). The success of this alternative interpretative scheme raises broader questions about the extent to which medicalisation of distress, via the diagnostic act, afflicts patients with the secondary, self-stigmatising effects of being labelled 'psychiatrically ill', and the extent to which this occurs not only for those diagnosed with 'schizophrenia' but for a whole host of behavioural and emotional difficulties currently captured by medical terms.

There is now ample research regarding the stigmatising effects of diagnostic labels (Purvis et al., 1988; Parle, 2012). For instance, we know that the most common public perception of 'mental disorder' is that it is biological in origin (Angermeyer & Matschinger 2005) – a perception that fuels stigma. For example, people believed to suffer from 'brain disorders' are treated more harshly than people believed to be suffering from social or psychological issues (Mehta, 1997) because people driven by biology are viewed as less free and predictable, and therefore more dangerous than 'ordinary people'. The application of the biomedical model to the realm of mental health has created fear in both sufferers and the public. As diagnosis therefore imports stigma-making meanings (in addition to foreclosing other more helpful interpretative alternatives), it can, as the case of Eleanor Longden illustrates, hinder more than enable the 'recovery' it aims to facilitate.

The fact is that medical language and meaning fuels stigma, and obliges us to accept the subtle ways in which the mental health professions drive stigma through their biological/diagnostic framing of emotional distress. Unfortunately, many professionals (as well as anti-stigma campaigns) remain oblivious to this contradiction: by continuing to use stigmatising medical language in their fight against stigma, they exacerbate the problem they purport to address.

CURRENT DIAGNOSTIC CATEGORIES ARE ANTI-SCIENCE

In April 2013 Thomas Insel, the previous president of the US-based National Institute of Mental Health (NIMH), the largest funding body for mental health research globally, declared that the 'NIMH will be re-orienting its research away from DSM categories ... [because of the DSM's] weakness is its lack of validity'. As he stated:

> DSM diagnoses are based on a consensus about clusters of clinical symptoms, not any objective laboratory measure. In the rest of medicine, this would be equivalent to creating diagnostic systems based on the nature of chest pain or the quality of fever. (Insel, 2013)

Insel suggests that neurobiological research has failed to discover biological markers not through want of trying, but because the disorders for which biomarkers are sought literally have no reality in our biology. They are rather the products of committees who gather periodically to define disorders by way of group consensus. While these processes and definitions may be interesting enough (to social scientists), they are no more likely to map on to neurobiological markers than are the speculative categories dreamed up by any group who predominately rely on an admixture of contradictory research and personal experience. For Insel, not only are our diagnostic systems inadequately constructed, they are also responsible for hampering neurobiological research. He states:

> I spent 13 years at NIMH really pushing on the neuroscience and genetics of mental disorders, and when I look back on that I realize that while I think I succeeded at getting lots of really cool papers published by cool scientists at fairly large costs—I think $20 billion—I don't think we moved the needle in reducing suicide, reducing hospitalizations, improving recovery for the tens of millions of people who have mental illness. (Insel in Rogers, 2017)

Our diagnostic systems have systematically misled research, which in turn has hobbled clinical outcomes. This is why, as Insel put it, 'we cannot succeed if we use

DSM categories as the "gold standard"' (Insel, 2013). Rather we should first aspire to find biomarkers and only then identify and name the corresponding symptom clusters as a given disorder. In this sense, Insel's position is not anti-diagnosis. It aims to provide a better basis for diagnosis and research. The diagnostic system that Insel proposes must therefore 'build up' from research data (genetic, imaging, physiologic and cognitive data), rather than seek to verify committee-contrived categories post hoc. Until the data is gathered, Insel believes we have no other choice than to deploy the DSM for clinical purposes, the assumption being that it is better to have a faulty diagnostic system than none at all.

While Insel's solution to the diagnostic crisis is not accepted by the majority of critics, what is interesting is what his solution presupposes: that the DSM has hindered neurobiological research because the diagnostic categories included are not rooted in any biological reality. This is to say – and to use my own words – because the separate disorders into which the DSM organised diverse behavioural and mental phenomena were largely the outcome of vote-based judgments settled by a small, culturally-homogenous subset of professionals who were socially positioned at a given time to have their judgments ratified by the American Psychiatric Association, they are social constructs that do not capture discrete patterns of biologically-rooted pathological feeling and behaviour identified by way of objective research processes (Davies, 2017).

To accept Insel's critique of our diagnostic systems is not necessarily to accept his solution, it is merely to agree that searching for markers for categories arrived at by way of committee consensus and voting is a scientifically futile exercise.

NIMH's decision to no longer fund projects based upon the DSM diagnoses raises another pertinent question: If the largest research organisation internationally for mental health research has lost confidence in our diagnostic nosologies, and for scientific good reason, why then should clinicians and service users continue to stake their professional and personal lives upon them? If our diagnostic systems have severely misled neurobiological research, why then do we not similarly discard them for misleading clinical practice?

FALSE PSYCHIATRIC EPIDEMICS

Our diagnostic manuals promote themselves as 'descriptive'. We have already explored why this is misleading, as diagnoses endow the experience they describe with medical meaning. A further reason why they are not purely descriptive is because psychiatric labels, once established, assume a social life of their own, that is, they are highly *proscriptive* social categories, in that they help shape and direct the forms suffering can take.

To illustrate this, consider the following. When a new diagnostic category arrives in DSM or ICD, incidence rates of the 'disorder' it describes regularly escalate. After ADHD entered the DSM in 1994 (having before been called ADD), incidence rates tripled by 2004. After self-harm was included in 1994, as a symptom of borderline personality disorder, rates doubled by the mid-2000s (Davies, 2013). And again, before dissociative personality disorder entered the DSM in 1980 there were about 200 related cases, a number that escalated to 40,000 by the year 2000 (Maldonado & Spiegal, 2008). After Asperger's was included in 1994, rates of autism increased twenty-fold by 2010. Finally, once Bipolar II was added in 2000, the ratio of bipolar verse unipolar depression doubled by 2010 (Davies, 2013).

What can account for these escalations? An obvious explanation is that once a disorder gains social recognition, doctors are more likely to look for it in patients, patients are more likely to look for it in themselves, and pharmaceutical companies are more likely to market the condition and the relevant drug interventions. Such factors are well documented and most certainly play a role in rising incidence rates. One factor receiving far less attention, however, is that once a new diagnostic category gains traction it becomes reified in our cultural imagination as a new expressive possibility. As a new disorder becomes known and ratified by a trusted authority, people begin to select that disorder, unawares, as a vehicle through which to manifest and communicate their distress (Davies, 2013).

This phenomenon belies the conventional view that diagnostic categories simply reflect 'psychopathology', capturing stable clinical syndromes that are broadly consistent across time and space. While this is the most common view of diagnosis, even a cursory reading of psychiatric history shows it to be naive at best (Paris, 2013). Within parameters, the behaviours and feelings these categories capture come and go, cluster and re-cluster into different configurations or 'syndromes', but more often the categories themselves can provide new scripts in terms of which suffering is unconsciously shaped and enacted.

Anthropologists have coined an opposite term for this scripting of suffering: 'mimesis'. This describes the process by which people unwittingly absorb and perform shared cultural scripts about how to act in order to achieve certain desired ends. It is well documented in the anthropological literature that mimesis regularly occurs in the performance of distress, enabling the communication of suffering through ways-of-being that are socially recognisable (Littlewood, 2001). In short, human beings seem to be invested with a developed capacity to mould bodily and mental experiences to the norms of their cultures, or, as Anne Harrington (2012) has put it, 'to learn the scripts about what kinds of things should be happening to them as they fall ill ... and then they literally embody them'. After all, it is crucial that we express our distress in ways that makes sense to the people around us otherwise we may end up not just ill, but ostracised (ibid.). Thus understood, the notion of mimesis is useful in explaining how the creation and ratification of new disorder categories can increase incidences of the very phenomena they purport to disinterestedly depict.

THE MAJOR DEFENCES OF DIAGNOSIS CAN BE EASILY COUNTERED

A useful way of addressing this issue will be to advance and address each of the main defences.

Without a diagnosis a person can't access care. Without labels millions would go untreated

Response: The fact that being medicalised is a precondition for receiving care highlights a systemic failing within our mental health services rather than a virtue of diagnosis. The solution to this problem is to de-medicalise services so diagnosis no longer needs to be a precondition.

Diagnosis aids our understanding of the 'patient' - the label informs us about the problem we are dealing with

Response: The opposite is just as likely true – a label often encourages oversight of a person's specificity and uniqueness, creating the illusion of understanding. It also misleads professionals and 'patients' by pathologising understandable human reactions, while reducing human complexity to a label that has no corresponding biological reality. Additionally, poor diagnostic reliability indicates that as any diagnosis is highly contestable it is also likely to mislead. Its main purpose is to resolve disagreement between professionals by converting a person's problem into a hypothetical 'disorder' about which both can agree.

Diagnostic categories facilitate research – without them there would be no agreement on what we are researching and no possibility of making generalisations

Response: Because the correspondence between diagnostic categories and the realities of either individual experience or biological reality is tenuous, these categories may mislead research. This is why the US National Institute of Mental Health will no longer fund research based on these categories.

Diagnosis brings recognition to groups of sufferers who would otherwise be ignored

Response: History and anthropology has taught us there are infinite ways of validating suffering that does not involve diagnosis and its associated implications. Furthermore, while the validation of suffering is important, so too is considering the nature of that validation. It is debatable whether diagnostic validation is less harmful than helpful given its many adverse effects.

We need diagnostic nomenclature in order to smoothly facilitate communication between professionals regarding the phenomena they purport to understand and treat

Response: There are alternative modes of communication that do not implicitly pathologise; for example, psychological formulation can be a trustworthy, useful and respectful way of facilitating communication.

Diagnoses are just helpful guides. We know they are not rooted in some biological substratum

Response: These labels hold great weight in society and for their recipients irrespective of the professional's particular philosophical position. Just because a label is ascribed with a healthy dose of uncertainty, it does not follow that it will be received in the same spirit. A diagnostic label is more powerful than the individual physician ascribing it, hence the comparative irrelevance of the physician's personal viewpoint.

CONCLUSION

Given the many problems with psychiatric diagnosis, and the contestable nature of the defending arguments, wide compliance with the diagnostic system may have less to do with clinical and academic considerations than with professional concerns about status, power, fear of marginalisation, the pragmatics of convenience and the perceived lack of viable alternatives. The current diagnostic crisis therefore emerges at the crossroads of two converging forces, the first being the adverse effects of diagnosis and over-medicalisation itself (and the contribution this makes to poor mental health) and the second being the systemic and professional interests and obligations that have made diagnosis the linchpin of mental health services.

The crisis therefore concerns what to do in the face of this dawning contradiction: how to diminish the influence of unhelpful forces in a system built entirely upon their assumed value and utility. While I would not presume to offer a complete answer to such a complex problem, I would venture that, at the very least, the four following shifts must occur if this contradiction is to be resolved in a direction favouring de-medicalisation. The first is that current and credible alternatives, such as psychological formulation, must gain evermore traction, moving from a peripheral to a central place in services. The second, and for purposes of research, is that we move towards developing a new non-medical nosology, one that does not pathologise or essentialise the styles of suffering people commonly manifest, while recognising that such styles are not fixed entities but change in response to shifting socio-cultural dynamics. Third, we move from a regulatory culture permitting commercial interests to expand and promote medicalisation towards regulation prohibiting such interests from having a role in shaping narratives or provision. Fourth, and to echo Kinderman (2014), we move mental health services away from being primarily hospital- and clinic-based to being community based – a move that will also entail a shift of power from individual clinicians to teams, from medical to non-medical approaches, and from professionals to service users.

6

MENTAL HEALTH IN CRISIS

Ron Roberts

> The language of the market colonizes ever new areas of experience, reaching in to what might have been regarded as the inviolable sanctuaries of the human heart. Do we not now talk of emotional investments, of the returns we get for our relationships?
>
> Seabrook, 1990: 12

CONTEXT AND KNOWLEDGE

In science as in life, context is everything. For matters of convenience, scientific studies often involve the attempt to isolate events and processes from their wider context. For giving us a handle on the complexity of the world, this has been a useful strategy. But it can also at times lead one astray – painting a picture of the world which is too simple and ignores obvious truths. Looking back after a lengthy career, Harvard psychologist Jerome Kagan (2012) bemoaned the fact that both academic and clinical branches of the discipline had too often been indifferent to the settings in which observations were made. He noted this was a problem not only in laboratory settings but intrinsic to the categorisation of mental disorders which takes no stock of the interpersonal environment and history of the person for whom problems have arisen.

If the side-lining of context has been a problematic feature of much behavioural science, it has also been characteristic of our understanding of science itself. In part this is not surprising, as science prides itself on attaining knowledge which is universally valid – true for all systems studied, no matter where or when. The assumption that this is possible has led to significant advances in our understanding of the non-biological world. Not so of course in the world of the social sciences, where obvious differences in culture, behaviour and beliefs are bound to particular places and times in human history.

This problem of context, however, extends beyond our ability to generate recognised truths about the human condition and situates itself also within the temple of knowledge itself. This means that our systems of knowledge as well as the content of that knowledge are context bound. Dreams of universal truth in actuality lie beyond the waking hours. Because we have been led by enlightenment values to aspire to universal knowledge, we have been blind to the fact that these values are tied to culture. I have argued elsewhere (Roberts, 2015) that the notion of objective universal truth (the Archimedean view from nowhere) – its value, power and utility notwithstanding – should be considered as tied to the normative beliefs of western imperial culture – and a particular subculture within that – principally, economically powerful, white males, who have for centuries occupied privileged and pivotal roles at the heart of political, economic, cultural and social life. The core of these beliefs holds that the maintenance of emotional and physical distance between investigator and investigated is essential to scientific method. This belief as a standard is perpetuated in part through the reproduction of existing power structures both in society at large and within the academic community every generation. In short, there is an uncanny resemblance between our ideas of truth (which stress universality, emotional neutrality and freedom from moral values) and the means by which those in power conduct themselves in the pursuit of personal, corporate and national profit.

One consequence of this unacknowledged interplay between scientific and political methods is that the social-economic and political framework within which science is conducted has largely escaped scrutiny. If we consider psychology in particular, its inception, historical development and emergence as a fully-fledged scientific enterprise have all been influenced by the structure and content of capitalist development. This is true with respect to the concepts it has employed, the type of methods used, the kinds of questions raised, the focus of these questions, and the nature of the answers given to these questions. I have discussed this argument in depth elsewhere (Roberts, 2015) but specific aspects of it are worth highlighting here, notably in regard to our current notions of mental health, disorder and illness and how we seek to address what we consider problematic in this domain.

PSYCHOLOGY AND CAPITALISM: IDEOLOGY

Before considering the associations between capitalist ideology and constructions of mental health, we should first say that there is barely an area of psychology which has not been touched by the invisible hand of market ideology: artificial intelligence, behaviourism, behavioural economics, biological psychology, cognitive science, decision science, educational psychology, evolutionary psychology, intelligence, occupational psychology, personality and social psychology to name but a few. What these have in common is that they assume as the starting point of enquiry, the validity of a decontextualised, de-historicised vision of the person that our alienated 'individuality' (Fromm, 1973) and social existence under capitalism can be ignored. These all preclude any possibility that the 'real life of the individual' can be 'understood as the interiorisation of political relations' (Sève, 1978: 2).

An important example of the deficiencies of such a perspective concerns free will, a key problem in contemporary neuroscience, which, following the mechanistic logic of capitalist thought, tags it as epiphenomenal to neural processes. In this scheme of things, we are not free and are not responsible for our actions. Cast adrift from historical thought, however, the neuroscientists are missing a trick. Even cherished notions of free will have their own history. In her off-modern excursion into this history, Svetlana Boym (2010) reminds us that our notion of free will derives from a tradition of public political debate began in the ancient Greek polis. As Greek democratic ideals waned, what had at first been a forum for public political freedom became internalised as an ideal. The Stoic notion of the 'inner polis' came into being, propounding a philosophy of 'inner freedom'. Freedom as such was no longer exercised in a public forum but in an interior theatre in which decisions were reached. With the decline of the public polis, it reappeared in the 'inner citadel of one's self' (2010: 85). Boym's reflections clearly show that the origin of free will does not reside in neural architecture.

This is a shining example of a more general problem in psychology's relationship to capitalism: it enacts what Boym (2001: 99) would call a 'charismatic concealment' of social relations by identifying social and historical processes as properties of individuals. As well as free will, memory, resilience, efficacy, attitudes, intelligence and health can all be considered properties of social systems. A necessary consequence of social, economic and political life subordinated to psychological (and bio-psychological) speculation is that social space becomes depoliticised. Psychological discourse, assuming individual weaknesses, vulnerabilities, defects and excesses then comes to inhabit space which was once reserved for political and moral debate. I encountered one of the more ludicrous examples of this at a conference on political psychology. Researchers seeking to explain anti-Semitism endeavoured to locate it in the cognitive structures and predispositions of individuals, a fruitless anti-historical strategy akin to studying original sin as a branch of social neuroscience!

By now the two advantages that mainstream psychological discourse offers to capitalism should be apparent. First of all, psychology offers capitalism an ideological get-out-of-jail-free card, as a crutch claiming the motivational structure in capitalist (exploitative) social relations are rooted in human nature whilst simultaneously providing a distraction from rigorous scrutiny of the system itself. After all, if capitalism, which has underpinned industrialisation, global trade, imperialism, apartheid, exploitation and war, is *not* taken to be a natural expression of our postulated inherently flawed nature, then a question regarding alternative arrangements for commerce and trade quickly arises.

The second favour that psychology bestows upon capitalism concerns the causal model it provides for explaining world events. If we subscribe to a view that the misfortunes of the world stem from the behaviour of aberrant individuals, we open doors to a doctrine of social control predicated on the necessity to maintain order by means of the constant surveillance of potentially dangerous/troublesome individuals. This 'psychocentric' culture may be considered a focal point in the genesis of social injustice in so far as it calls for individual rather than social reformation (Rimke, 2018). The ultimate expression of this in a totalitarian society is that everyone eventually falls under suspicion, deemed a potential risk to societal stability. However, before that point is reached the mental health system plays a key role in identifying who these miscreants may be and specifying ways in which they be dealt with and the threat reduced.

The relation between capitalism and psychology though is more than this. Psychology has not only provided cover for capitalist enterprise but has been shaped by it. Feeding on psychology's thirst, as a relatively young science, for recognition, acceptance and influence, it has been co-opted to help further the goals of states, corporations and businesses – frequently through assistance to the military. One of the first points of intersection between psychology's craving for scientific credibility and the state/corporate desire for power came with the imperative, during capitalism's early development, to categorise and count. What began life in the 18th century as political arithmetic – a tool to aid in the collection of economic and demographic data to facilitate economic and political planning (Roberts, 2015; Mazzucato, 2018) – eventually morphed into two distinct disciplines: statistics, which constituted the basis for scientific psychology, and economics. Under the rubric of behavioural economics and decision science, in the 21st century they are once again joined at the hip.

PSYCHOLOGY AND CAPITALISM: SURVEILLANCE

In late capitalist society, surveillance is fundamental to the workings of the economy. From the original panoptical form discussed by Foucault there have developed multiple divergent forms of being scrutinised by power. There are of course the ubiquitous CCTV cameras which patrol every nook and cranny of public space, at once converting it to corporate space. The perennial performance reviews and appraisals at work are another. Then there are the everyday digital spies which invade our computing machinery, from cookies keeping track of our movements through the World Wide Web to the big data deities of the information age, Facebook, Google and Amazon, crunching our data, to analyse, profile and sell on the free market.

To the above may be added self-surveillance, where we literally and figuratively seek to increase the happiness quotient of the world by changing how we look and feel about ourselves, aspiring via the never-ending purchase of consumer products and acts of self-promotion in cyberspace to be a 'model' of attraction. For this to be possible, our psyches must be conditioned to detect as imperfections any aspect of our existence which can be plausibly constructed as in need of financially mediated improvement. Less obvious than the above forms, there is the policing of our moods and emotional reactions by others; sales personnel and customer service representatives who, if not seeking to steer our emotional reactions towards a purchase, are forever sorry that we feel as we do about the products or services which have led us to complain, whilst never expressing penitence for their company or organisation's role in the genesis of our dissatisfaction – what Adams (2016: 7) refers to as the 'reactive management of consumer expectations'. If we can't be happy, the customer service goal is that we be at least 'satisfied', and if we are not satisfied then those on the other end of the phone must feign being truly, madly sorry for *our feelings* – regret not for their misdemeanours but for the existence of our feelings in the midst of the corporate play. The faceless scriptwriters who compose the business end of these exchanges prefer a form of psychic numbing to their indifference – an emotional state familiar to consumers of psychiatric drugs. The similarity is not accidental. Emotional labour in the service economy should be understood as both the faking of emotions by workers to promote business transactions and the manipulation of our emotions through their labour, even when conducted remotely as with the manufacture and prescribing of mood regulators.

To complete the trinity of psychological and capitalist relations, we may speak of the linguistic surveillance and takeover of our inner and social lives; the colonisation of all facets of human existence in terms of the language and logic of the market so that everything may now be spoken of in terms of investments, transactions and commodities. Years before we were engulfed by the financial crisis, Seabrook (1990: 12) wrote of the psychological catastrophe that rampant capitalism had already achieved: 'The bottom line has invaded the recesses of our personal lives [...] and we all have our price.' Our psychological make up is now not only constituted de facto under capitalism, but a major reason why capitalism is able to continue when it has long ago been placed on life support.

MENTAL HEALTH, CAPITALISM AND CULTURE

Examining the intertwined nature of psychology and capitalism and understanding how the former functions on behalf of the latter to depoliticise events and mystify the source of human troubles is no mere academic debate. Immense practical consequences flow from this symbiotic dance of destruction. The customary grounds for moral and political debate – human conflict, troubling passions and unequal power dynamics – were long ago surrendered to bio-psychiatric hegemony in the mental health industry. The venom that greeted the maverick Scottish psychiatrist Ronnie Laing for suggesting that disturbed behaviour could be comprehended in human and political terms outside the realms of bio-psychiatric speculation was (and remains) indicative of precisely what professional sins were being revealed.

To grasp the nature of the Faustian pact between the mental health industry and organised power necessitates deliberation on the concept of mental health itself. Accustomed as we are to using it, we easily forget that it is not a value-free conceptual entity, nor does it provide a neutral or natural description of how human minds work. Szasz (1961) has been the most prominent critic to insist that ideas of mental health and illness embody value judgments about what is or is not acceptable or desirable to do, think and feel. In Arendt's lectures on Kant's political philosophy, we are reminded that the validity of judgements per se 'never have the validity of cognitive or scientific propositions' (Arendt, 1978: 269); they are, accordingly, matters of taste with which nobody can be compelled to agree. Hence the decision as to whether one uses the concept or not is a philosophical, political or ideological choice. It is also a historical one.

In line with this argument, numerous commentators have pointed to the variability in standards, interpretations and meanings ascribed to behaviour and experience across cultures. Such work has been of value in demonstrating psychiatry's lax adherence to scientific standards of measurement and construct validity (Davies, 2013) and in showing the cultural intelligibility of human responses to adversity across BAME ethnic cultures, responses which when subject to the power of the medical magic wand are transformed into indicators of psychiatric 'illness' (Littlewood and Lipsedge, 1997). Cross-cultural work has also been of value in international comparisons of recovery rates from forms of psychological distress. Several major studies of this type have been conducted (WHO, 1973; Jablensky et al., 1992; Bhugra, 2006). All show the same results: recovery rates from serious mental illnesses are superior in developing countries where fewer psychiatric services exist. For less serious problems (e.g. depression), data suggest that problems are greatest in North America and least in Africa.

Two main suggestions have been proposed to account for these findings: that better levels of social support exist in developing countries, and the possibility that psychiatric medication hinders recovery. Both may be influential. Little data exist on support whilst the contention that psychiatric medication is detrimental to recovery is well supported. Moncrief (2009) reviewed the findings of several which show that, even within western settings, psychiatric service users who avoid neuroleptic drugs do better than those who use them. One implication of these studies is that expansion of western-type psychiatric services into developing countries poses a clear and present danger to the people there. Careful evaluation of the reform programmes being instituted in developing countries such as China (Liu et al., 2011) following 'international advocacy', and WHO policy recommendations for 'internationally agreed and recognised standards in mental health service provision' (p. 215) will no doubt provide further test material. The reforms currently underway there can be said to comprise a third wave of western intervention, subsequent to the introduction of 'mental health institutions' by western missionaries in the 19th century, and the modernisation programmes of Deng Xiaoping which saw Western models of treatment and rehabilitation introduced. There are few grounds for optimism. The Chinese Society of Psychiatrists has been accused of complicity in the oppression of political and religious dissidents, using diagnoses such as 'political maniacs' or 'delusions of reform' alongside compulsory detention.

The political abuse of psychiatry has a long ignoble history (van Voren, 2010) and was a characteristic feature of the Soviet and Nazi periods. Less well known was that it became co-opted by the Argentine Junta during the 1970s and 1980s. Ramos (2013: 272) describes how within Argentine psychiatric circles 'membership in leftist organizations was counted as evidence of mental illness' and during the first year of General Videla's military dictatorship, the editor of one journal (*Neuropsichiatria*) 'dedicated the journal to the fight against subversion.' As in the UK, the press endorsed the psychiatric stance favoured by state authorities and utilised psychiatric theory to pathologise subversives. Van Voren (2010: 34) argues that psychiatrists within these repressive systems were 'probably unaware that they engaged in unethical behavior and ... were part of a governmental repressive machinery.' That is a generous judgement. It is easy to overlook these as historical curiosities from which the West has little to learn. However, examples of collaboration between repressive governmental agencies and mainstream mental health professions can be found closer to home. In the UK the intertwined activities of the Department for Work and Pensions (DWP), the US insurance giant Unum and the Centre for Psychosocial and Disability Research at Cardiff University which it sponsored for over 6 years, provide a case in point. The company states that the bio-psycho-social model of disability has taken pride of place in 'its approach to medical underwriting'. This approach, inspired by behavioural economics, has been employed to justify sanctioning disabled people and denying them benefits. The catastrophic effects of this on people's mental and physical well-being has been detailed in a harrowing report by Mehta et al. (2018). The British Medical Association (BMA) and the British Psychological Society (BPS) condemned these assessments, but a number of lessons for practitioners and researchers remain. These include the by now well-established observation that states and corporations may use ideologically inflected research to further inhumane policy objectives. Van Voren makes a further telling comment that we would do well to ponder:

> Admittedly, those involved in the struggle against political abuse of psychiatry never reached full consensus on what the exact boundaries were between political abuse of psychiatry and more general misuse of psychiatric practice. (2010: 35)

Szasz (2004: xiii) was convinced that the boundary between them was non-existent, that institutional psychiatry always 'serves the interests of the coercers' and that any recognition of this is taboo. Similarly, the place of behavioural economics in the pantheon of abuse also remains taboo. Space precludes a more detailed examination of this thesis. But complicity with the ideological employment of behavioural science by the powerful and the facts of legally sanctioned compulsory psychiatric detention and treatment in many western countries as well as the distant historical outposts of the Gulag should give us no cause for complacency. The distinguished historian of psychiatry, Roy Porter (2002: 217) offered no crumbs of comfort in questioning whether the repertoire of psychiatric treatments dispensed in the second half of the 20th century had actually become more humane, or more firmly based in 'rationality and sanity'. In an era when global politics once again marches to the drumbeats of fascism, complacency, in a context in which mainstream psychiatry has operated as a debate free zone, would be foolhardy.

Where cross-cultural psychiatry has undoubtedly fallen down is in failing to extend the principles of cultural intelligibility beyond the confines of their black and ethnic minority (BME) patients: presuming the cultural, historical and hermeneutic homogeneity of all their ethnic *majority* patients, across lines of class, gender and disability is a weakness, laying the profession open to accusations of racism by positioning the mental ill-health of ethnic minorities alone as open to cultural interpretation. In this way the mental health of BME patients is constructed as an exotic object and the white subject remains simultaneously indivisible and invisible. The function of this, no doubt, is to preserve the self-proclaimed universal legitimacy of western psychiatry methods. It is this legitimacy that Summerfield (2017: 11) attacks. His argument is worth repeating. 'Diagnoses,' he says, 'are merely descriptive constructions, conceptual devices, and are drawn up by us, not by nature.' This means that 'mental disorder' posited as an 'entity essentially lying outside situation, society, and culture, which is identifiable anywhere using a common [western] methodology' is not valid. He continues:

> 'depression' has no exact equivalent in non-Western cultures ... because these do not share a Western ethnopsychology that defines 'emotion' as internal, often biological, unintentioned, distinct from cognition and a feature of individuals rather than situations. (2017: 11)

It is not, and cannot therefore be true that 'depression' exists as a universal concept.

What strikes one as strange, if one pursues this cross-cultural line of thought, is how the complex value judgments surrounding mental health are taken as articles of faith in scientific psychiatry. But in truth the phrase 'scientific psychiatry' is practically an oxymoron supported only by the medical profession, the political class and the media, an unholy constellation of allegiances who ought to raise doubts regarding the veracity of what is being asserted by them. Szasz (2008) remained adamant that their assertions were lies. Davies' (2013) anthropological exploration of the workings of institutional psychiatry and its sacred text, the DSM – worthy of inclusion in any 'dissenting histories of the present' (Boym, 2017: 32) – exposes the circus whereby Big Pharma money, desires for profit, prestige and status, scientific pretence and skulduggery, occupational bullying and career threats to dissenting voices coalesce to give us the grand lie of pharmaceutically treatable, biologically-based mental illnesses. All this is politically expedient and legally permissible for reasons outlined above.

We are entitled to ask whether the role of the profit motive in mental health care would continue to hold sway without the willing aid of a supine media and a cohort of journalists supplying the glue of celebrity endorsement of mental health 'conditions'. The self-proclaimed liberal press is possibly the worst offender. In 2002, the *Guardian* newspaper received five million dollars from the Gates Foundation to promote both health and development issues, a year in which the Gates Foundation itself, set up by Microsoft's former boss, bought shares in Big Pharma to the value of $205 million (Bank & Buckman, 2002). The paper regularly publishes articles about mental health. In *Capitalism on Campus* (Roberts, 2018: 109) I subjected a group of these to further analysis. Around half were opinion pieces, almost entirely uncritical and rehearsed previously challenged views on the efficacy and mode of action of psychiatric drugs. In one, Mark Brown (2017) stated that a recent 'mega-analysis' had answered 'once and for all' the question of whether anti-depressants work. He went on to declare that 'depression was an "illness"', that 'anti-depressant efficacy was now established' and that the research in question had found 'a clinically significant positive difference in people's mood when they were given the SSRI rather than a placebo'. In reality the study concerned (Hieronymus et al., 2017) had not made this claim.

More recently (February 2018) in response to a study of anti-depressant efficacy (Cipriani et al., 2018) the paper ran an article by health editor Sarah Boseley (2018) headlined 'The drugs do work: antidepressants are effective, study shows'. This uncritical piece, containing supportive comments from several psychiatrists, was accompanied on the same day by a further credulous offering from editor Mark Rice-Oxley (2018) exhorting us to 'get on with taking and prescribing them' as it is 'official' that 'they work'. It is important to note that none of the numerous critiques of psychiatric medication and its associated tainted science has ever been given 'official' status by the paper, a fact which speaks volumes about the influence of Big Pharma. The original article was savaged a couple of days later by Joanna Moncrieff, Hugh Middleton and John Read in correspondence to the paper (*Guardian*, 2018a) in which it was pointed out that '"real world" studies show that people treated with antidepressants have poor outcomes and fare worse than depressed people who do not receive antidepressants. Increased prescribing will do more harm than good'.

Embarrassed but not shamed, the paper responded two days later with a piece by Rhik Samadder (2018) again telling us that 'anti-depressants work'. Samadder tells us, in all seriousness, that he knows this because 'half the people I know are on them'. The following day (28 February) Rhiannon Lucy-Costlett (2018) kept up the barrage to 'say with certainty that anti-depressants are effective drugs'. According to Lucy-Costlett, 'treating your depression is like learning your times tables'. Several days later, another collection of letters appeared, this time from psychiatrists and various satisfied users declaring that 'Antidepressants work – and we are the proof' (*Guardian*, 2018b). The collection was given a more prominent placing on the website than the aforementioned professional scepticism of Moncrieff, Middleton and Read. A mere three days passed by before its sister paper the *Observer* published yet another article, also on the *Guardian* website, from Alice Gibbs (2018), with a headline pleading with us to believe – as if we didn't know by now – that 'Anti-depressants do work'. The ubiquity with which the same phrase was churned out suggests a disturbing lack of imagination at one of the UK's best papers. Why that should be the case is open to speculation. An alternative hypothesis – the lack of a good thesaurus at Guardian HQ – doesn't hold water in the digital age.

There are evident ethical problems to consider when large numbers of a newspaper's journalists, many of whom declare a history of anti-depressant medication, none of whom are scientifically qualified to assess relevant evidence, are given free rein to tell readers unequivocally that they work, when there exists a serious body of dissenting scientific literature which is given almost no space. Any troubling aspects of this seem to have flown under the paper's radar, along with any nuanced understanding of the concept of proof. The *Guardian* has clearly understood the value of repetition in stultifying the brains of its readers, as well as the value of the money it receives from its backers. Its readers, however, have no inkling of what lies behind its persistent attempts to shape not only what they think but also which mind-altering pharmaceutical substances they should imbibe for the good of their mental health. To discuss the issue of funding and how it relates to content is proscribed in the online (and printed) spaces devoted to readers' comments, as is anything which contemplates, suggests or implies that the *Guardian* may be biased. That plausible hypothesis, they inform its readers, is 'against our community standards'. The online version of the paper's daily pleading with its readers for financial support comes with the claim that its journalism 'free from commercial bias' enables them to 'give a voice to the voiceless, challenge the powerful and hold them to account'. Any small print providing an exemption to Big Pharma was omitted. The newspaper's owners understand capitalism well. Not only in where to secure a few shillings from rich backers but in how to hide unpalatable truths and sell the myth of mental-health liberalism to readers. How the not so 'liberal' right-wing press cover 'mental health' issues is a task I'll leave to others, but it is hard not to conclude that the press has an unquestioned and unquestionable faith in both the universality of mental illness and the appropriateness of dealing with it via psychiatric drugs. This does not serve democracy well.

MENTAL HEALTH BEYOND THE CAPITALIST CRISIS

We began this chapter discussing the importance of context. If we accept that the current crises in mental health – with respect to both the incidence and prevalence of distress and the troubling nature of psychiatric interventions – is an integral aspect of the interlinked local and global crises tied to modern capitalism, the question arises as to what kinds of future scenarios we can imagine for both if capitalism does not last. A few years ago, the question would have seemed fanciful.

Once the Berlin wall had come down, Fukuyama (1992) declared the triumph of western liberal democracy as a form of governance inextricably tied to the supremacy of capitalist-free markets. Fukuyama's thesis of the 'end of history', an expression of Western hubris, was not greeted with universal acclaim, and with the benefit of hindsight seems hopelessly flawed. The resurgence of Russia and China as global powers, the financial crisis of 2008, the growth of xenophobia, nostalgia for authoritarian and fascist forms of rule are a clear signal that the forces of history do not go gentle into that good night, while the marriage of convenience between democracy and capitalism already has. Perhaps the most significant aspect of the changing world, however, is a growing consensus, even in economic and sociological circles (Wallerstein et al., 2013; Streeck, 2016), that capitalism is living on borrowed time – that a period of historical transformation is looming which may cast aside the once cast-iron certainties of indefinite survival for a system predicated on the perpetual creation of crisis.

The question at this critical juncture is whether political intervention is capable of saving capitalism from itself. The efficacy of the post-World War Two remedial systems for parking debt and warding off systemic collapse – Keynesian stimulation, state and privately accumulated debt – have been serially exhausted. The reforming toolbag is empty, and that is before one considers the role of information technology, artificial intelligence and the 'rise of the robots' (Ford, 2015) changing the face of labour exploitation forever (Mason, 2015), or indeed the ultimate contradiction between a system premised on infinite expansion meeting the reality of dwindling natural resources and ecosystem collapse. Almost all that remains in keeping capitalism's sinking ship afloat is psychological: belief that there is no viable alternative, a failure of imagination and courage in political leaders, and the very resilience of people to neoliberalism contributing to the resilience of neoliberalism – our continually adjusting to it rather than abandoning it. On the other hand, what could contribute to its final demise is also psychological: the distrust of key market players that the system can be restored to health and the dawning realisation that there is little left to commodify. Once the psyche has been colonised and distributed to shareholders, what is left? The progressive demise of the capitalist system has opened the way for a period of 'deep indeterminacy' (Streeck, 2016: 12) which may presage – in the absence of the emergence of viable alternatives – a period of global anarchy, economic stagnation, corruption and oligarchic inequality. These are enormous threats to human well-being.

As this demise gains traction, one can expect commerce to take a nostalgic turn, endlessly recycling and reselling an imagined past or the imagined futures of the past – a kind of phantom capitalism hoping to prop itself up by the strength of what no longer exists. In the fog generated by the slow death of capitalism, however, one can discern the slow birth of the future in the various alternative guises in which human living is already being reimagined: ecological awareness, renewable energy, sustainable living, intersectionality, multiculturalism, the renaissance of feminism, Black Lives Matter and the end of medicalised mental health. Resistance to these is considerable, yet they contain the seeds of a brighter more responsible future that envisions our material, social and psychological lives under a different, more just umbrella. 'The need for a less suicidal political economy', Streeck (2016: 251) stressed, 'is urgent'. Mazzucato (2018) added that we must strive to make it one in which value creation, not extraction, is given the highest regard. At our best and with belief, heart and organisation, our preparations for the future can succeed.

7

EXISTENTIAL CRISIS

Joel Vos

Imagine you visit the doctor after injuring your toe, and the doctor suggests removing your tonsils as a cure. This would be called a medical error. Imagine now, that you are underfed because you live from the food bank, and that you have infections due to the mould in your flat. Imagine that you tell your doctor that you are worried about your physical and mental health due to your socio-economic disenfranchisement. And imagine that in response the doctor recommends you improve your way of thinking, or take antidepressants. You would call this a psychotherapeutic error. The doctor has identified the wrong cause of your worries. Your problem is not that you have an unrealistic way of thinking but that you are confronted with real socio-economic problems. Learning to think differently may help you cope better, but whatever mindset you have will not change the physical reality you are confronted with. There is an existential reality which you cannot 'cure' or deny, one that will always feel raw. This is life. One may argue that any psychological or psychiatric treatment that does not take this into account is unrealistic and normative-oppressive in nature. Any 'cure' that tells you that you need to change while you are confronted with life's unchangeable facts may burden you with a sense of guilt for something that you can never be fundamentally responsible for.

However, mental health services that are offered in western countries predominantly offer therapies that focus on the individual. Since 2014, the UK has even been offering CBT to unemployed people in job centres. Governmental rules dictate that those who do not exhibit a positive outlook must undergo reprogramming or otherwise risk losing benefits. There is an existential reality which cannot be denied, but which may get little attention in such Orwellian programmes. Problems are individualised by offering a variety of standard therapies. Research shows that these treatments have limited effects, whereas therapies that directly address the existential reality may have larger effects for individuals confronted with life's boundaries (Vos, 2018). Of course, it may be expected that most therapists will be nuanced and will not rigidly impose unrealistic expectations on their clients. However, several researchers have suggested there may be an implicit culture of blaming clients for their unchosen life circumstances. This may be called a 'meritocratic fallacy' – that an individual's competencies and efforts totally determine their life situation, and consequently that if anything goes wrong people have only themselves to blame.

A SOCIAL-EXISTENTIAL PERSPECTIVE

The journalist Barbara Ehrenreich (2010) describes how we live in a 'smile-or-die' culture where we are not allowed to feel sad or frustrated about our existential reality. She describes how she felt that she was not only sick because she had cancer, but had a second disease which was not thinking positively about having cancer. She describes how she began to see this disease of positive thinking everywhere she looked. For example, the jobless person not only felt bad about being jobless, they also felt bad about feeling bad. This unrealistic culture of positive psychology creates extra internal pressure in already psychologically difficult situations. Mental health care workers contribute to this culture when searching for personal causes and solutions, even when a client is confronted with an undeniably hard reality. This alienation from one's own existential feelings may come at the cost of existential crisis and mental health problems.

An existential crisis is a crisis in someone's existence: something that seems to challenge or undermine their life. When a doctor tells you that you only have a couple of weeks left to live, your life is literally at stake, and it is natural that you experience an existential crisis. An existential crisis is more fundamental than a psychological crisis, although both types of crises often go hand in hand (Vos, 2018). In a psychological crisis, you could still realise that as long as you experience good physical health and are not dying, you may still find solutions to your problems, such as learning new psychological skills to cope better with your problems. However, in an existential crisis you are confronted not merely with your psychological capability or your lack thereof, but also with the limitations of the *human condition*. You realise that all humans are limited and will die, and that you are no exception to this rule. Everything you do in life may start to look mundane and superficial in this light. You may have been worried about your appearance at a friend's party, but this becomes futile when examined from the perspective of life and death. Why would you waste your limited time and money on buying the latest phone when you cannot take this into your grave? Research indicates that a majority of people when confronted with hard, undeniable limitations in life (e.g. war, poverty or life-threatening disease) ask such existential questions. Their main request for help is: 'How can I live a meaningful and satisfying life despite life's challenges?' (Vos, 2016).

As Ehrenreich indicated, mental health problems may be caused by the expectations we have about life, what we find meaningful and what standards we set for ourselves – and these expectations can be manipulated by governments, corporations and social media. For example, in the past, governments would explicitly command 'thou shalt work' or the Bank of England would implicitly command 'thou shalt buy' by lowering interest rates. However, such external interventions are relatively non-specific and one can to a degree escape them. To control citizens more, governments can impose stricter measures and punishments, such as threats to remove benefits for the slightest infraction of rules. However, control is more effective when individuals discipline themselves. Foucault (2012) describes how the exercise of such internal authority has replaced that of external authorities. People start to govern themselves. We instruct ourselves that it is not good to be without work or the latest gadget, and accordingly feel bad when we are unemployed or empty-pocketed. So we internalise messages from external sources which seek to direct our lifestyles.

We are officially free, but are continuously bombarded by advertisements and messages from social media. An average person in London is exposed to over 4,000 commercials and logos per day. These societal messages influence the standards we have about life and how we think about ourselves. Therefore not only do our external socio-economic circumstances make us feel stressed or frustrated when we lose benefits, but we also change internally and frustrate ourselves by the expectations we set for our life. In the past an unemployed individual would be told to 'get a job', but the jobless person could psychologically put this message aside and not let their self-image be determined by this. However, nowadays an additional implicit message is given by newspapers, social media, tweeting ministers or presidents: 'If you do not get a job, you are a loser and you only have yourself to blame.' In our meritocratic era, success and failure are attributed to someone's actions, ignoring the realities of societal and existential complexities. An individual may develop mental health problems, not merely because the loss of employment can be stressful but because they also feel guilty and bad about themselves. The complexity of work situations and economic conjunctures gets reduced to self-blame.

Therefore our expectations about how we should live and the standards that we set for ourselves are strongly determined by others. Individuals often think of themselves as unique and self-determining, but in reality, lifestyle decisions are often influenced by the wider social context. However, traditional therapies often pay little attention to such existential problems, and may even exacerbate psychological problems by explicitly or implicitly searching for the cause of psychological problems and solutions in the client instead of doing justice to their complex social reality: 'It is not society that causes the problems, and I do not have a problem, I am the problem myself.'

THE ECONOMIC SYSTEM IS NOT VALUE-NEUTRAL

Many critical theorists (e.g. from the Frankfurt School) have analysed how our current economic system comes with a one-dimensional vision (Marcuse, 1964), for instance by focusing on acquiring materialistic objects and having quantifiable success. New capitalism brings a culture which implicitly and explicitly influences how we think about what is meaningful in life. Meanings such as happiness, health, beauty and conserving the planet have no structural place in economics (Schumacher, 1973). The current economic system has created a narrow focus on specific types of meaning concerned with identity, happiness and consumption, as William Davies (2015) demonstrates in his book *The Happiness Industry*. However, meaning is a more comprehensive concept (Vos, 2018). Not all our actions are driven by identity creation, having nice experiences or being happy. They can be driven by other meaningful motivations such as helping others, belonging to a community, fighting for justice, or religious belief. So economics is not neutral and has become an end in itself instead of merely being a means to 'the good life', as Skidelsky and Skidelsky (2013) describe in their book with the much-telling title *How Much is Enough: Money and the Good Life.*

Although modern economic theories idealise the idea of freedom (e.g. the free market of supply and demand), in reality this freedom can be frightening on a psychological level. In his book *Escape from Freedom*, Fromm (1941/2011) described how individuals try to escape from freedom. What Fromm described is pertinent today. Conformist individuals change their ideal self to conform to a perception of society's preferred type of personality, and thus may lose what they personally find meaningful in the process. They govern themselves on the basis of explicit and implicit expectations that they have absorbed from their social context. Another way to escape from freedom is by delegating the decisions and control of ourselves to others, for instance by voting for authoritarian leaders – evidenced in the 'creeping fascism and the rise of the far right' in the US and Europe (Faulkner & Dhati, 2017). Also, individuals may attempt to destroy the world as it is in a desperate attempt to save themself from being crushed by fear of the world (e.g. by destroying the climate). In line with research from sociologists, it may be argued that modern capitalism actually stimulates all three forms of escape instead of realising the formal ideology of freedom (Vos, 2019).

THE CAPITALIST LIFE SYNDROME

What is the mental health impact of our current economic system with its specific ideas about how we should live our lives? The answer to this question may be summarised as the 'capitalist life syndrome' (Vos, 2019). This comprises six phenomena.

First, individuals suffering from the capitalist life syndrome live in a capitalist society. This means that they live in an economic system which focuses on private ownership, profit, and a free and competitive market. This not only regulates economic relationships between people, but also our self-perceptions. People are taught from childhood onwards to live life to the max and optimise their economic function, as they need to achieve the highest in their education, career, salary, family life, housing, luxury goods and so on. Becoming yourself, contributing to the well-being of others or fighting for justice have relatively little value in this model. Instead, economists tell us, self-interest and competition are the cornerstones of economic prosperity.

Second, research with 45,000 individuals from all continents reveals that those living in capitalist countries focus more on superficial meanings than those in other countries (Vos, 2019). They seek meaning primarily in materialism, hedonism or themselves. They concentrate on buying things, achieving success in their career, improving social status, maximising pleasure, or developing themselves to the max. In contrast, they focus less on social connections, altruism or higher purposes such as creating a just society or following a religious calling. This research also shows a strong relationship between having superficial meanings in life and lower psychological and physical well-being. That is, individuals who dominantly focus on materialistic, hedonic and self-oriented meanings in life experience more mental health problems such as depression and anxiety. This explains the frequently reported happiness paradox in capitalist societies: individuals report being happy, but this doesn't necessarily mean a deep sense of fulfilment.

Third, some capitalist authors promote a functionalist approach to life. Stereotypically formulated, they believe that they can simply demand or buy meaning in life, like any materialistic product on the market. They feel their desire for meaning can be quickly fulfilled, like buying a 'Burger McMeaning' (Vos, 2018). For instance, they expect life fulfilment by going on foreign holidays, binge-drinking or taking drugs. Although these McMeanings might deliver temporary satisfaction, they do not provide a deeper sense of meaningfulness in life. An extreme example can be found in the assertion by Becker, an economist, that all economic behaviour can be explained by the ability to increase economic utility or efficiency (Becker, 1992). This includes love, which according to him means that people derive utility from each other. In other words, Becker writes that meaning is about a relationship that increases each other's well-being. This implies that love would disappear if one partner would no longer be able to increase the other's well-being, for instance because of physical or mental health problems. This utilitarian approach has made love vulnerable to manipulation and commercial exploitation, such as Hollywood movies, Valentine business, dating shows on TV, and dating websites which tell us that true love can be ordered like a burger. Research shows that love is, of course, for most people much more complex than this.

Fourth, individuals identify themselves with their capitalist lifestyle, consciously or unconsciously. They may believe that this lifestyle is the best they can achieve in life. They may even passionately defend the capitalist system, even when this doesn't help them to realise what they experience as meaningful in life. They do not see – or do not want to see – the violence and manipulation of their perceptions and values. Therefore, the term 'capitalist life syndrome' is derived from a pseudo-psychological diagnosis called the 'Stockholm syndrome' (Vos, 2019). This syndrome was first described in a psychological analysis of the positive feelings that hostages felt towards their captors during a violent bank robbery in Stockholm in

1973. The Stockholm syndrome describes the condition that causes hostages to develop a psychological allegiance with their captors. Despite the actual danger that the captors are to their well-being, hostages develop positive feelings towards them, and even refuse to co-operate with the police or legal system. The hostages believe in the humanity of their hostage-takers, and that they hold the same values. Similarly, individuals in capitalist societies often vote for people who do not act in their interests. This explains the electoral paradox that political scientists struggle to understand. Many in difficult socio-economic circumstances endorse policies that will factually decrease their own opportunities, for instance by voting for policies of austerity, benefit cuts, lower taxes for corporations and high-earners, or voting for Brexit and seeing EU funding for their deprived region cut.

Fifth, the capitalist life is also associated with structural existential crises. Surveys indicate that many feel fundamentally anxious and uncertain about life, suffer from indecision, feel inauthentic, and are driven by an existential urgency to get the most out of life (Vos, 2018, 2019). Similar to the Stockholm hostages, individuals suffer from capitalist fatalism. That is, they feel a lack of mastery over their lives, stuck in their life situation with no alternative. This fatalism is created by the socio-economic power structures within which individuals are embedded, for example the low likelihood of a woman growing up on a council estate reaching a top position in a major corporation. The fatalism is also caused by one's own expectations that the capitalist dream (e.g. getting that perfect job) is their only option. Fatalism fulfils a crucial role in maintaining the economic system, as people feel they have no other option than finding meaning in the market of working and buying. The sense of freedom is narrowed. Consequently, when confronted with freedom beyond their current position in the system (e.g. due to long-term unemployment or structural discrimination) many feel existentially lost.

Sixth, the capitalist life syndrome has an immediate impact on mental and physical well-being. This does not necessarily entail that someone has clinical depression or anxiety, but rather feel a structural sense of emotional discomfort, unhappiness or lack of satisfaction in life: 'I cannot put my finger on it, but ...'. Research shows that a focus on superficial types of meaning and the sense of fatalism often lead to low quality of life (Vos, 2018, 2019). Although individuals may live for a long time with such feelings, they may ultimately experience an existential crisis. In general, research shows that the more capitalistic characteristics a country has, the more mental health problems individuals have (e.g. Skidelsky & Skidelsky, 2013).

DISCUSSION

This chapter warns against the psychotherapeutic error of automatically personalising mental health problems. Instead, the individual's existential and socio-economic reality should be examined. Such holistic assessment would focus on recovery instead of cure. The traditional medical perspective suggests that mental health care workers try to cure someone's problems by searching for an ultimate personal cause and a matching solution (e.g. learning better psychological techniques or taking psychopharmacological drugs). Numerous studies show that individuals do not ask for mental health support to get personally cured. They wish to live a meaningful and satisfying life despite their personal and socio-economic circumstances. To help someone recover means that they are helped to achieve this meaning-oriented goal.

It has been argued that all effective mental health treatments help clients to live a more meaningful life (Vos, 2018). Clients do not change simply because they follow a practitioner's instructions, but because they are motivated to change: change is meaningful. A review of hundreds of clinical trials revealed that the more explicit and systematic mental health treatments address questions about existence and meaning, the more effective they are (Vos, 2018). Examples of such effective psychological therapies are existential and meaning-centred therapy (Vos, 2016). Despite an overwhelming evidence-base for their effectiveness, these treatments play a minimum role in national mental health services.

This implies the willingness of practitioners to examine their own role, and to accept the possibility that they are contributing to clients' problems, for instance by personalising the causes of existential and socio-economic realities. Practitioners can reflect on how their treatment coerces individuals to fit an unjust system, instead of acknowledging their real struggle and empowering them to transform that struggle into a society-transforming attitude. Acknowledging the existential reality therefore goes beyond therapy rooms, into the wider world (Vos, 2018).

8

CRISIS IN ACADEMIA

Ron Roberts

RECENT HISTORY: A NEOLIBERAL MAKEOVER

In the showbusiness world it has been said that years pass before one becomes an overnight sensation. Both the current crisis in student mental health and the decline in the credibility and purpose of the academy have enjoyed a similarly long gestation. Arguably, they have similar roots.

The tale begins in the late 1970s. The nefarious transformation of education's tools of 'freedom and opportunity' into 'sources of indignity' (Back, 2016: 81) is a direct, inevitable product of Margaret Thatcher's policy goal to introduce 'market discipline' into higher education. The focus of the Iron Lady's desire was to position students at the heart of a repurposed economic engine propelling institutions of learning into compliance with corporate governance. Her reign saw the British economy refashioned in a manner faithful to the principles espoused by the Chicago school of economists. The birth of the neoliberal project following these principles – and with it, disaster capitalism (Klein, 2007) – occurred first in Chile, in a calculated brutal fashion, via the CIA-sponsored removal of Salvador Allende's democratically elected government.

As part of Thatcher's ideological vision, a new model army of students were 'expected to serve as the personification of market pressures' (Furedi, 2011: 3). Necessary to this upheaval was the commodification of learning. From year-long programmes of study into bite-sized purchasable packages of knowledge, the UK system imported modularisation from the US. With the creation of the student as consumer, measures were put in place designed to ease money from students' (and parents') pockets. (See Roberts, 2018, for a fuller timetable of these changes.) The timeline began with the introduction of full tuition fees for foreign students in 1981, followed by freezing and then reducing the student grant. The introduction of loans followed. A key moment was the Dearing Report (National Committee of Inquiry into Higher Education, 1997), which recommended students pay 25% of the cost of tuition. Tuition fees, set at £1,000 per year, arrived a year later. Five years later, the new Labour Government increased these to £3,000 and in 2012 under the Liberal–Tory coalition government they were raised to £9,000. The introduction and increases in fees occurred despite protestations by Tony Blair (Labour) that 'Labour has no plans to introduce tuition fees'. They were described by leaders of the other main parties as 'one of the most pernicious political acts' (Charles Kennedy: Liberal Party) and 'a tax on learning' (Iain Duncan Smith: Conservative). All three parties eventually argued that there was no alternative – a view premised on rejecting education as a social good for all. Under the new status quo, education became a privileged product to be paid for not only by those who could afford it, but also by those who enjoyed it; a resource now imagined as a component of one's personal capital portfolio.

The elimination of maintenance grants and the introduction of tuition fees were accompanied by a raft of 'disciplinary' marketing instruments designed to change the behaviour of staff and students. The first of these was the Research Assessment Exercise (RAE) in 1986, followed by the Teaching Quality Assessment (TQA) in 1992, and the National Student Survey (NSS) in 2005. The RAE mutated into the Research Excellence Framework (REF) in 2014 and the TQA was exhumed and recast as the Teaching Excellence Framework (TEF) in 2017. The latter has effectively reframed university education as something akin to an Olympic sport in which 'successful' institutions can be 'awarded' Gold, Silver or Bronze ratings. Together, the above funding changes and the creation of an obsessive measurement culture fundamentally changed universities. What were once primarily seats of learning and knowledge are now, at heart, enterprises for generating profit.

The crisis we are embedded within is a direct and unavoidable consequence of the neoliberal remaking of education and the violence it has wrought on staff and students. It has facilitated the corrosive branding of British universities; witness endless pointless mission statements, websites overrun with 'badges, stickers and logos' (Scott, 2017) and much gobbledygook – the higher education version of Newspeak, about 'enhancing' the 'student experience'. Like Orwell's original in *1984*, the current wave of educational discourse functions to suppress independent thought, with academic freedom disappearing in the slipstream. As in Huxley's *Brave New World*, it promotes the pleasure principle as the apex of human achievement – high National Student Survey (NSS) scores as the ultimate university accomplishment.

The community most at ease in the contemporary higher education dystopia is an administrative cohort, described by Evans (2004: 3) as 'bureaucratic Rottweilers ... snapping at all our heels'. The (mis)selling of university education – 'expensive, overhyped and a con' (Chakrabortty, 2018) – has brought us to a situation in which the paranoid dystopian musings of sci-fi doyen Philip K. Dick now provide a descriptive fit to the life of learning in late capitalism. In one of his novels, Dick (2014) renamed educational institutions as 'Lies Incorporated'. A university education, once the field of life-long dreams, is now, like most neoliberal institutions, a breeding ground for corruption and scandal: Vice-Chancellors' expenses and severance packages (Mosher, 1998); mismanagement (Baker, 2011) and resignations (Hodges, 2009a); NSS scores (BBC News Online, 2008); reporting of student numbers (Hodges, 2009b); student enrolment (*Telegraph*, 2012); promotion (Baker, 2011); validation practices (BBC News Online, 2011); misleading marketing (Busby, 2018); sexual harassment (Devlin & Marsh, 2018); and sexual violence against female students (Turner, 2017). These are just a few to have graced the pages of the British press – a single chapter would not be sufficient to capture how widespread the malaise on campus is. Many scandals remain hidden. The list above, however, is suggestive of the workings of a banana republic, of the unchecked entitlements of privilege and the desperation to maintain an institution's corporate image.

A recent case in the UK concerning the physical assault of a female student at Sussex University (Turner, 2017) exemplifies how university management privileges image reputation over students' well-being. An investigation spurred by reports in the *Independent* newspaper (Pells, 2017) and conducted by Nicole Westmarland, a leading researcher on domestic violence, criticised the HR department for prioritising the attacker's protection and the university's reputation over student safety. That the university's conduct followed the publication a year earlier of a Universities UK report into sexual violence and harassment – itself criticised as 'inadequate' (Weale & Batty, 2016) – gives further evidence of the priorities of university management.

As surely as the lugubrious influence of money binds management, accountants and advertisers together in a nexus of power, disinformation, lethargy and corruption, it alienates and perplexes staff and instructs students to embrace a different set of values – with all their attendant costs. We will now examine what has happened to both staff and student mental health in this same period.

MENTAL HEALTH ON CAMPUS

The political and economic restructuring of higher education in the UK parallels that observed throughout continental Europe. In part, this has been a response to the perceived need for universities to function as partners in the transformation and restructuring of global capital markets. In this vision higher education serves as the research and development arm of the corporate world. In this role universities have been required to increase the proportion of graduates in the population, providing a ready source of highly skilled labour at home equipped to deal with the technological demands of emerging knowledge-based economies. Thus, a major role of the universities is to supply in abundance – excess even – the intellectual labour needed to enhance economic competitiveness.

The philosophy supporting this reimagining of higher education is enshrined in the Lisbon declaration of the European University Association (2007). This called for a greater role for private finance in setting the strategic aims of universities. One irony of the Lisbon declaration is that while it called for greater autonomy and diversity on the part of universities, the consequence has been the opposite: a stultified bureaucratic and business-friendly agenda. Tucker (2012) provides a damning indictment of this mode of production. The factories of learning – the dark satanic mills of the 21st century (Roberts, 2018) – are now run by managers who follow a model 'that resembles the late Soviet model of industry during the Brezhnev era' (Tucker, 2012: 102). Tucker describes this managerial class as 'failed academics and clerical and secretarial staff' (p. 108). The psychological dynamics of economic and bureaucratic stagnation that characterised the late Soviet era are now reproduced in the apathy, disbelief and failed belief that colonises the minds of staff and students on campus. The assault on academic reality and the mental health of academy workers has been long, slow and deliberate. Drawing on Baudrillard's conception of the simulacrum, Roberts and Hewer (2015) consider the burgeoning unreality of academic life as a direct challenge to mental health. They depict a toxic environment in which the usual signifiers of scholarly life connote nothing beyond their role in representing the façade of university life. This is the ivory tower unmasked as a Potemkin village. They write:

> One might assume that the academic hierarchy is highly qualified, that lecturers teach and carry out meaningful research while students study, engage in debate and take exams. The physical geographical infrastructure including libraries, computers and lecture halls in conjunction with the espousal of values, an institutional history and the roll call of illustrious alumni adds to the sense of belief in the 'reality' of the institution and one's place within it. The internalisation of these relationships, artefacts and institutional history forms a basis for the belief that the university is 'real'. However, what if the image fails to map reality? What if professors do not hold high academic qualifications or are not leaders in their field? What if principles of meritocracy are abandoned in favour of other political or social criteria? (2015: 175–6).

The neoliberal tsunami reconstructing the function and meaning of the university at the behest of corporate elites has left in its wake a hollowed-out shell in which staff, left in the ruins to fend for themselves, increasingly casualised, wander aimlessly in search of meaning. The bureaucratic and misanthropic chicanery that constitutes everyday life has led the sharpest minds to conclude that a love of money exceeds any love for knowledge. Not surprisingly, accusations of bullying have multiplied, prompting concerns 'that a culture of harassment and intimidation is thriving in Britain's leading universities', where 'career sabotage' is not unusual and 'HR managers appear more concerned about avoiding negative publicity than protecting staff' (Devlin & Marsh, 2018). What psychological effect the UK's exodus from the EU will throw into this indigestible mix can only be imagined, but the effect on staff morale is unlikely to be positive. Already, prospects for international collaborations and funding have been compromised, so too the recruitment of academic and health service staff and students from Europe, as the country bathes in an increasingly racist light (Fazackerley, 2018). Universities are already expected to function as would-be checkpoints in the UK's toxic immigration system, with predictable unpleasant consequences. The looming burdens imposed by a post-Brexit visa landscape suggest that the omens for a smooth transition to the future are not good.

If cries from the campus suggest a dismal and unjust life for academics, what about the students, whose years of study are now nurtured under the watchful eye of managers parroting the corporate mission to 'enhance the student experience'? A good deal of evidence indicates things are no better here. Work detailing mental health difficulties and financial difficulties in populations of students began emerging in the 1990s. One of these (Roberts et al., 1999) noted even then that the mental health of students was, in general, poorer compared to the population norms for people of comparable age and gender. Poorer mental health was linked to the emerging norms of student economic life – longer working hours outside of study and difficulty paying bills. These findings have been corroborated in several studies since (e.g. Cooke et al., 2004; Carney et al., 2005). None of this should be considered surprising. The results of a meta-analysis by Richardson et al. (2013) of the relationship between debt and physical and mental health confirms that financial difficulties are implicated in poor mental health. Their findings evidenced significant relationships between debt and mental disorder, depression, suicide, problem drinking, drug dependence, neurotic and psychotic disorder. Much of the work has been cross-sectional, leaving some uncertainty in how to interpret causality in these relationships. However, evidence has emerged in more robust longitudinal studies linking financial difficulties with subsequent depression (Richardson et al., 2017) and an increased risk of later psychosis (Richardson et al., 2018).

Indebtedness in students has risen markedly alongside tuition fee increases, from £4,800 in 1997 (Swanton, 1997) to over £50,000 today (Institute of Fiscal Studies, 2017). Running parallel to students' worsening financial predicament is a rise in student engagement in the sex industry, as financially stressed students seek to cash-in their 'sexual capital' as sources of well-paid employment run dry, debts escalate and time to study is compressed by the need to find well-paid work to survive. The phenomenon has been observed across Europe (Duvall Smith, 2006), Australasia (Lantz, 2004) as well as the UK (Roberts et al., 2013; Sanders & Hardy, 2015), with research repeatedly pointing to debt and financial pressures as the driving force behind it. Recent research by Sagar et al. (2016) estimates that around 5% of the student population have engaged in work in the adult entertainment and sex industries.

It is hard not to conclude that policies at both the governmental and university level have contributed to poor student mental health. Figures from the Institute for Public Policy Research (IPPR) (2017) point to an increase of almost 500% in the disclosure of mental health conditions by students over a ten-year period, with significant increases in the demand for counselling and disability services. The report's authors, in line with previous work, conclude that students today experience lower well-being than young adults as a whole, and exhibit lower well-being than was previously the case. Information on student suicides provides further evidence. Data from the Office for National Statistics (2018) point to an underlying upward trend (see Figure 8.1 below).

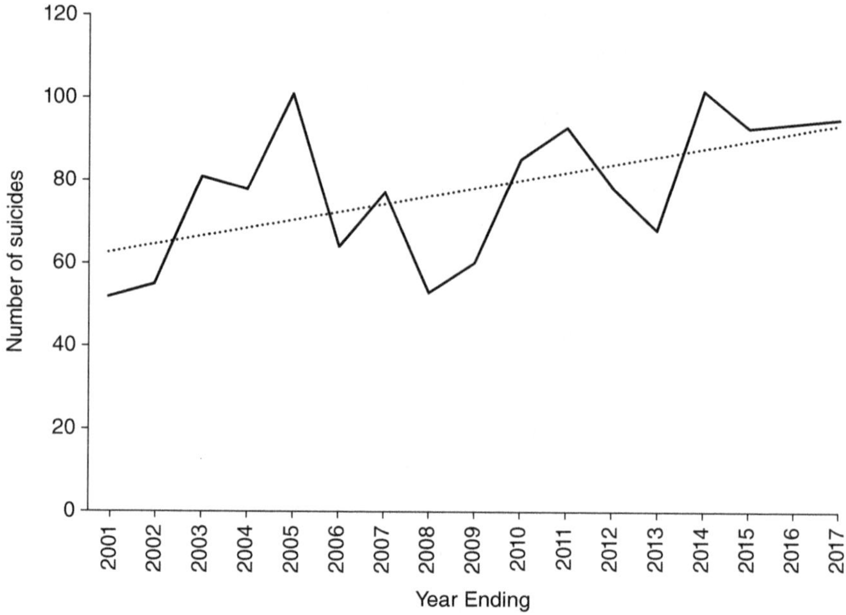

Figure 8.1 Number of higher education student suicides by year in England and Wales (adapted from Office for National Statistics, 2018)

The suicide rate amongst UK students is actually significantly lower (4.7 per 100,000) than in the general population of similar ages (Office for National Statistics, 2018). That ought to provide no grounds for comfort given the acknowledged better material and social circumstances of students compared to the wider population. Increased rates are in fact found for students from lower socio-economic backgrounds. The IPPR report contends that the major driving forces behind deteriorating mental health are academic demands, the pressure to obtain a good degree as well as social and financial pressures. It is notable that study demands have been cited by over 70% of students (YouGov, 2016) as a primary source of stress. This data warrants reflection within a broader context.

A glimpse of what that broader context is comes from statistics that show a 50% increase in the number of under-18s admitted to hospital from self-harm between 2009/10 and 2014/15 (Gilburt, 2016). These are the prime years in a period of government-imposed austerity. The 'mental health epidemic' in young people (Kalia, 2018) may tell us more about the state of society than individual resilience. We live in times when central government has unleashed a full-scale assault on social and welfare provision, including cuts to community mental health services and education funding and created a relentless and draconian culture of testing in schools. And beyond the classroom and the lecture theatre awaits the precarious world of work, with the gig economy, unpaid internships, zero-hours contracts and few well-paid jobs. Within this broader canvas there can be no doubt that the meaning and value of a 'good education' has changed. Tertiary level study is now more stressful, not because it is more difficult than 20 years ago but because the context within which it occurs has undergone a radical brutalising change. That context is now experienced as more demanding, first of all because an increasingly prescriptive education system no longer prepares or nurtures an independent approach to learning and secondly because the meaning of education itself has been overhauled; it is now less intrinsically valued and more often than not seen as a lifeline and a staging post to survival in the dog-eat-dog neoliberal world.

Corroborating evidence comes from one of the few robust analyses of National Student Survey (NSS) scores. This concluded that students' satisfaction ratings should not be used as a method of ranking as the scores are in large part markers, not of the quality of education but for students' 'readiness and confidence to face the labour market' (Lenton, 2015: 126–7). Our understanding of the crisis in student mental health then, needs to move away both from labelling them as 'snowflakes' and from deliberations about the difficulty of higher education. This is a generation that has been targeted to pay the price for the folly of those who precipitated the financial crisis. One might hope that given this, universities would be keen to reassess what is actually going on; be keen to examine the extent to which it bears at least a sliver of responsibility for the well-being of those who study and work on their grounds; and be ready to adopt a more challenging stance to government policy.

PSYCHOLOGICAL GOVERNANCE: THE POLITICS OF MENTAL HEALTH

One cannot hope to understand how universities have responded to this crisis without contemplating the role of psychological discourse (and its management) in the post-industrial landscape. The most recent phase of capitalism has been marked by a dependence not just on emotional labour but on forms of psychological governance that seek to mould, configure, influence and control the cognitive and affective contours of life. Psychological governance understood as 'attempts to advance, manage and regulate the social good through targeting the minds of individuals as a means of changing their behaviour' (Gillies & Edwards, 2017: 96) is now a core strategy in the management toolbox. Parker (2014b) provides an instructive discussion of how female middle management have been employed to stifle discontent in the academic workplace. In addition to this it is now predominantly university bureaucrats untrained in any mental health discipline who sanction exemptions and extensions to course work and course deadlines on mental health grounds. Official recording of these invariably involves the diagnostic labelling of students with no acknowledgement of the questionable reliability or validity of these. This signals a new development in the turf wars between psychology and psychiatry and de facto renders university bureaucrats as (undercover) agents of psychiatry.

The corporate management of workers' and students' moods signifies a decisive change in the role of psychological knowledge in the economic system. Psychology, a willing accomplice to capitalism almost since its inception (Roberts, 2015), has, under neoliberalism, seen its language decoupled from the discipline and appropriated by states and corporations seeking greater control and compliance over both the workforce and the population. We will consider here two key aspects of this.

First, with little critical attention, the issue of 'psychological vulnerability' has become weaponised and now constitutes a battleground whereby critical forces seeking to ameliorate the consequences of neoliberalism meet, head-on, state and corporate forces seeking to impose and prioritise that vulnerability as a condition of control. This is increasingly played out in an expressed concern with student mental health. Barely a week goes by without an email appearing in my inbox from various policy forums inviting attendees to cough up money to attend conferences led by people who for years have exhibited no discernible interest in student mental health. Often the specified tasks for these gatherings include 'strategies for reducing stigma' and 'improving awareness of mental health' along with how to implement the latest 'mental health strategy'. Universities UK provide a case in point on their website, declaring that higher education leaders are 'adopting mental health as a strategic imperative'. If one was judging the meaning of this sentence by the effect of management practices on the mood of academic staff, one would have to conclude that it was poor mental health that was being prioritised. Notwithstanding this reality,

'Professor Steve West, Chair, Universities UK Mental Health in Higher Education Working Group' goes on to make the 'case for action', which comprises four reasons why 'mental health should be a strategic priority'. These include dealing with the 'demand for and costs of student support services' which are said to be 'increasing sharply', facilitating a 'positive impact on student retention and engagement' and 'increased satisfaction' by which is probably meant NSS scores. At the top of the list is the 'risk' arising from a 'narrative of crisis in student well-being and mental health' (Universities UK, 2018). In summary, the priority is to contain a dangerous narrative, reduce costs and boost NSS scores. On the basis of these statements, if one wants to find evidence of a genuine and concerted desire to improve young people's well-being one should look elsewhere.

The similarity in the discursive referents employed (e.g. well-being, good mental health and appropriate support) by those with a genuine interest and concern with student well-being and by those merely seeking a competitive (marketing) advantage, either for their institutions or themselves personally, means that one must interpret initiatives carefully. A danger is that this concern will prop up the supremacy of the management status quo in universities as well as increasingly discredited psychiatric models of distress, not only in regard to the labels used to categorise distress but also the ideas about the underlying reasons for that distress.

A genuine desire to address the crisis in young people's mental health must perforce deal with questions of justice and the structural nature of the causes of injustice. The IPPR highlighted a marked difference in mental health problems by gender. In 16–24-year-olds, 28% of women were found to experience mental health problems (predominantly 'depression', 'anxiety' and self-harm), compared to 10% of men. The report makes no attempt to explain this. Such a marked difference is difficult to explain on any other basis than the daily insults, harassment, assaults and injustices which women undergo and the systematic pressures to conform to societal expectations – which include keeping quiet about how they are treated. Justice, however, is an issue that is notable by its absence from anything Universities UK, the British government or individual universities with exhortations of 'positive thinking' and 'inspirational talk' have to say. The record of universities when it comes to violence against women, as previously stated, is lamentable. Only when the protection of student well-being comes ahead of protecting the 'reputation' and image of establishments will there be a chance of effectively dealing with the mental health crisis.

Any strategic campaign for positive mental health that doesn't come out in favour of abolishing tuition fees, restoring the maintenance grant, ending austerity, providing meaningful and well-paid work for young people, ending the culture of testing in primary and secondary education, ending cuts in community mental health services and actively seeking to promote a culture of safety for women cannot be taken seriously.

Promotion of better 'mental health' would be more fruitful if it came with a critique of how constructions of mental health – notably diagnoses and labelling – whether by self or other, function in a wider politics of consciousness (Clements & Davies, 2013). As discussed in Chapter 5, the pantheon of mental disorders is largely a corporate construction, sponsored by pharmaceutical companies with a vested interest in medicalising human suffering. The status quo construction of individual vulnerability that forms the backdrop to the majority of mental health campaigns plays into the hands of the economic, corporate and professional forces which promote the existential (psychiatric) categories that need to be replaced. When institutional campaigns, such as those promoted by Universities UK, talk of 'raising awareness' all too often they can be read as attempts to exclude avenues of critical thought from consideration. Research consistently shows that stigma (fear and prejudice) against 'mental illness' is related to media depictions of insanity and to the continued dominance of the biomedical model of distress that feeds these (Read et al., 2013). Attempts at 'mental health literacy' predicated on the notion of mental illness as (biologically-based) illness like any other, merely fan the flames. Read and colleagues reviewed 22 correlational studies, spanning 35 years and 14 countries. In these, belief in biogenetic causal models was repeatedly associated with negative attitudes toward and desire for social distance from the 'mentally ill'. Similarly, belief in psychosocial causation of distress was associated with positive attitudes. Psychiatric labels as well as beliefs about causation have similarly been shown to have negative consequences. When one considers that psychiatrists largely subscribe to biological models of causation whilst the general public attach more importance to social and environmental factors, one can readily discern the dangers posed by mental health literacy and awareness campaigns.

The customary model of psychiatric disorder actively promotes the internalisation of identities of fragility, weaponises emotional display and undermines the self-confidence of people who seek help for their mental health (Furedi,

2016). The alternative is to cultivate forms of social and political support that build resilience. Identifying as a 'mental health system survivor' or a survivor of trauma and mistreatment is a more effective and empowering rhetorical resource than any identity built on being 'mentally ill' or 'disordered'. Whilst language pertaining to distress cannot avoid connotations of vulnerability, what it can do is reframe the meaning of that vulnerability in a way that it ceases to be construed as a lack, a persistent and enduring 'deficit' or defect – whether biochemical or genetic – which resides within an individual, absorbing and assuming an impersonal and uncontrollable responsibility for the social, economic and political sins of the world. It is regrettably the 'deficit model' that flourishes on campus – a case of putative chemical imbalances which favour corporate bank balances – and one which stands to benefit from official campaigns; it enshrines a commitment to promoting forms of vulnerability that assist state and corporate bodies, and which discount our capacity to challenge the powerful and change the world. Eccleston and Hayes contend that it is

> a diminished image of human potential [which] opens up people's emotions to assessment by the state and encourages dependence on ritualised forms of emotional support offered by state agencies … [It] replaces education with the social engineering of emotionally literate citizens who are also coached to experience emotional well-being. (2009: 135–6)

We must then distinguish a radical reconstruction of human vulnerability rooted in the inescapable contingencies of social acts and the workings of nature from a corporate construction of mental health. Actual mental well-being and 'corporate mental health' are at odds. The corporate view privatises the sources of stress (Fisher, 2009), pigeonholes people into pharmaceutically sponsored psychiatric categorises, assumes rather than discusses what constitutes well-being and delegitimizes justifiable protest, anger, outrage, anguish and despair. The latter are outlawed from organisational and state prescriptions of the happy citizen, who, it is deemed, must follow the edicts of positive psychology and accept whatever 'treatment' is given. The undertone to the conventional model of mental health care is that its subjects know their place and accept it without struggle.

The growth in mental health problems in young people in recent years is better understood not as an index of personal failure but as a consequence of ruthless economic policy decisions that have seen cuts in investment, training and job opportunities for young people, low wages, exorbitant loans and tuition fees, cuts to health and welfare services, a housing crisis as well as a savage school system where endemic testing reigns. To these multiple failures to invest in young people can be added the normalisation of exploitative advertising and marketing which uses the bodies and images of young people to sell dreams of unattainable lifestyles, property and wealth. The higher education industry as presently constituted is a net contributor to this conveyor belt of impossible aspirations.

The ongoing crises in academia are indicative of a broader malaise – one tied to an increasingly failed model of economic activity and its related norms of social governance. The attempts of the higher education branch of the global management elite to shore up the edifice of toxic neoliberalism, by their nature constitute quintessentially hostile acts. Kelly (1955: 510) postulated hostility as the 'continued effort to extort validational evidence in favour of a type of social prediction which has already proved itself a failure.' What we do about this system failure is the responsibility of us all.

9

THE ORGANISATIONAL CRISIS IN MENTAL HEALTH

Joel Vos

THE MATRIX OF MENTAL HEALTH IN CRISIS

Previous chapters paint a dim picture of the mental health system. We have seen how mental health problems are personalised, though it is often the structured social context that causes or exacerbates psychological problems, for instance via neo-colonialism, austerity measures and benefit cuts. The dominant economic system in western countries, capitalism, deeply affects social relationships, the academic world and individual well-being. Meanwhile, the care offered for mental health difficulties is predicated on diagnostic labels and psychopharmaceutical treatments which are not well supported by evidence. In the UK, national mental health care policy appears to be determined by a small coterie of influential voices with service users, mental health advocates and professionals marginalised.

What connects these trends? Several authors have called this the 'McDonaldisation' of mental health care (Binnie, 2015). But from where has this drawn its power? Is this because we have become addicted to consumption of on-demand products (Kunneman, 2005)? Do we live in times of social disintegration, impulsivity and meaninglessness which we attempt to keep at bay with pharmaceutical drugs and therapies providing quick fixes? Or do these cultural trends arise from the nature of our economic system and the deliberate intentions of corporations? Has capitalism become the final stage of human development, penetrating our minds and health care (Fukuyama,1992)? Do we therefore live in 'end times' in which everything is political, as the regulatory institutions and commercial interests shape our behaviour and experiences (Zizek, 2011)? Is our consent for this system manufactured by propaganda from corporate-owned media, advertising and think tanks, which shape our thinking to reflect implicit corporate priorities and interests (Herman & Chomsky, 1994)? Have academics contributed to this system by selling-out (Chomsky, 1967)?

In this era of mass manipulation, it seems difficult to distinguish fact from fiction. In this chapter we explore five possible explanations for the crises in mental health and the care system. These explanations are not independent; they may co-exist or interact to create the mental health realities discussed in this book.

GOVERNMENTAL POWERLESSNESS

Chapter 3 showed how McDonaldisation, silencing voices, structural bias and neo-colonialism influence how governments allocate mental health budgets. Why do policy makers and politicians behave in this manner? The most innocent answer would contend that they don't know any better. For instance, politicians who supported the launch and initial organisational design of the IAPT initiative (e.g. Ed Miliband and Gordon Brown) were not mental health experts. They depended on their advisers, most of whom had professional and personal interests in lobbying for IAPT. There may also have been a sense of impotence, stemming from insufficient information in a context where they had to urgently tackle widespread poor mental health and limited access to care. It may also have been a simple case of powerlessness, with lobbyists from the psychopharmaceutical industry and CBT so strong that their judgment was unduly influenced. Similarly, in African and Southeast-Asian countries, western psychiatrists are amongst those who offer advice and services to policy makers.

One perspective is that policy making has been infiltrated by corporate lobbying. There is evidence of biased media campaigns to promote CBT and IAPT (Rogers, 2009). In the US, direct-to-consumer drug advertising is permitted, exerting pressure on lay people to consider whether they suffer from similar ailments to those depicted. They may consult family doctors or pharmacists for treatment. Although this direct advertising can raise awareness of undiagnosed problems, there is evidence that these campaigns are detrimental to public health (Ventola, 2011). Drug companies employ many tactics to influence policies: funding research, pro-drug patient and carer-groups and advertising or disease promotion campaigns to the general public (Moncrieff, 2003). These tactics led Loren Mosher (1998) to resign as president of the American Psychiatric Association. In his letter of resignation, he wrote:

> Psychiatry has been almost completely bought out by the drug companies ... psychiatrists have become minions of drug company promotors ... No longer do we try to understand the whole person in their total context ... We condone and promote the widespread use and misuse of toxic chemicals that we know have serious long-term effects.

THE WEAKNESS OF THE POLITICAL LEFT

It can be argued that neoliberal ideas have colonised mental health care because of insufficient political opposition. The NHS has been restructured on neoliberal values under successive governments. Critics such as Jeremy Corbyn have argued that New Labour policies did not represent core left-wing values. Activists on the radical left argue that the left's weakness is a result of watering-down revolutionary demands to meet social-democratic aspirations, leaving space for vested corporate interests to be promoted. Others argue that the systems of power function as an intricate web in which well-meaning politicians are easily trapped. Politicians also often bring 'friends' from their former education, the media and the military (Jones, 2016). It has been argued, for example, that the Clintons had left-leaning policies before entering the White House, but were quickly corrupted by the plethora of advisers and the inertia of governmental departments (Lerner, 2006).

One could argue that left-wing ideologies have structurally ignored the mind. Marxists stress the determination of mental life by material conditions, and direct their campaigns toward seizure of the means of production and redressing inequalities in work space, housing and food distribution. Culture and mind have traditionally been regarded as entirely caused by material conditions. As we have seen, adverse material conditions do impact on the mind, and a just mental health care system should certainly address the unequal distribution of material working and living conditions. However, reality is more complex than a simple Marxist account conveys: the mind may be considered as an independent domain that also influences people's mental health and attitudes. Mass media has considerable influence on how people think about their life situation and politics.

The noted economist, John-Maynard Keynes, erred in his prediction that in our era we would work fewer hours with more wealth (Skidelsky, 2003). His error flowed from his assumption that people's desires were stable. During the 20th century, however, individuals sought to increase their living standards by buying expensive technological and other leisure products, with many of their desires directly manipulated by marketing (Skidelsky & Skidelsky, 2013). The short shrift given to the psychological domain in left theories may well have created a vacuum which corporations and neoliberal ideologists have willingly occupied. Consequently, the wars of the future may be played over our mind as much as material resources (Roberts, 2015). The means of mass manipulation matter just as much as the means of mass production.

THE SHOCK DOCTRINE OF MENTAL HEALTH CARE

We have suggested that politicians and policy makers are too receptive to lobbyists. However, the biased budget allocation could also be the consequence of an active strategy to transform mental health care in a manner conducive to the smooth functioning of the capitalistic system. For example, a number of British Secretaries of State for Health and Social Care have expressed an intention to privatise health care.

There is clear evidence that IAPT is congruent with capitalistic values. Treatments are selected and funded on the basis of cost-effectiveness, not the subjective experiences of service users. Service providers are evaluated and remunerated on the basis of payment-by-results and performance indicators. Similarly, the WHO (2003) has suggested that countries develop mental health systems that focus on payment-by-results. Therapists describe how they are under constant management pressure to achieve targets with an excessive workload and inadequate staffing and support. Furthermore, the UK Health and Social Care Act 2012 explicitly extended a market-based approach to the NHS, emphasising a diverse provider market, competition and patient choice as ways of improving health care. Several professional bodies have complained that little transparency exists over the outsourcing of mental health services; between 5% and 10% of all mental health services in the UK are privatised and Capita, Virgin, Accenture, Reed, G4S and Serco are lining up for lucrative contracts despite a minimal track record. There is also a trend towards treating people with mental health problems as 'consumers', for instance by experimenting with personal health budgets that consumers can use wherever they want (Forder et al., 2012).

These trends must be seen in the light of the dismantling and privatisation of the NHS (El-Gingihy, 2018).

The claim of 'innocence' offered in the previous section therefore cannot explain why the UK government has cut mental health funding. Of course, it is possible that this is connected to NHS budget deficits and austerity measures. However, a more critical hypothesis is that the mental health system is being set up for failure so that services can be subsequently privatised. As Chomsky (2011) has said:

> That's the standard technique of privatization: defund, make sure things don't work, people get angry, you hand it over to private capital. That's the Social Security scam. If they can succeed in defunding it – they've been trying for decades.

Another strategy used to privatise public services is to use a financial or economic crisis, or large-scale emergency that creates a public sense of shock, as an opportunity for restructuring. Naomi Klein (2007) called this strategy 'the shock doctrine'. In a similar way, budget cuts in mental health care are repackaged and used to sell ideas about 'efficiency savings' and 'reorganisation'. Under cover of the financial crisis, political advisors have sought to refashion health services as more outcome-oriented and privatised (McDaid & Knapp, 2010). Several countries have used austerity as an argument for the accelerated reorganisation of mental health services (e.g. Wahlbeck & McDaid, 2012). These decisions seem to be based on a small number of highly hypothetical and ideological reports and articles promoting the shock doctrine in mental health care:

> During the period of austerity that we now face, the National Health Service (NHS), including mental health services, will have to make efficiency savings at a time when demand for services is likely to rise. [...] Many potential areas for efficiency savings, such as resources invested in management and administration, are relevant ... The economic downturn may, however, also present a specific opportunity for radical innovation within the mental health system. (McDaid & Knapp, 2010)

SUCCESSES AND FAILURES OF HUMAN RIGHTS

Until relatively recently there was little care for those we would now regard as being mentally ill. The earlier impetus was to protect society from 'lunatics'. However, from the 17th century onwards, religious asylums and madhouses were founded, the latter being places where doctors experimented with treatments. Until the mid-20th century, individuals were frequently incarcerated, experimented upon or exterminated – as in Nazi Germany or the USSR under Stalin. The Universal Declaration of Human Rights (UDHR) in 1948 changed the situation in many countries (United Nations, 1948). Signatory countries agreed to protect the rights of citizens including those with mental problems. The WHO has been promoting a human rights perspective in global mental health care, seeking to oppose discrimination, misuse of power and unjustified hospitalisation and encourage the development of more humane care.

The WHO (2017) Mental Health Atlas shows that approximately two-thirds of all countries have laws to protect the rights of mentally ill individuals. However, only half of all countries conduct regular independent inspections of mental health facilities. In one-fifth of all countries, individuals must pay for their own care and for psychiatric drugs. There is considerable international variation in the numbers of mental health workers per 100,000 people. In Europe there are 50, in America 10, in Africa just one and Asia, three. In Europe and North America care is focused in the community, while elsewhere it is largely centralised in mental hospitals. The Atlas shows that whilst the human rights of mental health service users has improved in many countries, much remains to be done.

At first glance, the intention to legally safeguard vulnerable individuals seems positive, but the crucial question is how human rights are applied in practice (Gostin & Gable, 2004). A consortium of user-led organisations, allies and individual campaigners, led by the National Survivor User Network (www.nsun.org.uk), concluded that the British government structurally refuses to give people with mental health diagnoses full human rights as detailed in the United Nations Convention on the Rights of Persons with Disabilities (UNCRPD), and ignores voices from service users in their formal mental health care reviews. The UK Mental Health Act 1983 and Mental Capacity Act 2005 directly violates UDHR articles which state that 'everyone is entitled to all the rights and freedoms' and that 'no one shall be subjected to arbitrary detention or exile' (Lawton-Smith et al., 2008). Presently people can be forced to receive assessment and treatment in hospitals or in the community when experts judge they are a danger to themselves or others. False positives, where individuals are wrongly deemed incapable, are common. It has been argued that coercive practices may result from lack of skills, financial constraints or inadequate time to develop more equal and empowering relationships with patients (Stanford et al., 2017). Furthermore, the right to a fair trial for those with mental health problems has been called into question. Research shows they experience bias, lack support and frequently remain unaware of legal avenues of redress (IOPC, 2018). Several studies show how isolation and physical restraints are frequently used in care, leading to psychological deterioration and suicides (LeDeR, 2017). Use of restraint has significantly increased and at least 40 people have died 'in barbaric circumstances' (Kelso, 2018). Additionally, both access to mental health care and the length of waiting lists have been criticised by health advocates. So practices frequently fail to meet human rights standards.

Some commentators argue that human rights have been commodified, that attention has become focused on how well the service does – in terms of 'customer satisfaction' – rather than examining what service users really need (Moyn, 2018). In this guise human rights become a marketable service, open to celebrity endorsement, organisational branding and other marketing techniques. Under the shadow of neoliberalism, governments express a willingness to fulfil citizens' basic needs only as long as this doesn't interfere with the aims and desires of the wealthy. The result is a socio-economic environment that structurally undermines people's mental health. The human rights movement has often seen rights as a panacea, without realising the limitations of its aims. So governments offer minimum mental health care to maintain a supply of emotionally stable workers for the labour force. Mental health inherently depends on positive freedom, as problems are not only caused by failures to protect human rights. A lack of emancipation and empowerment and adverse socio-economic conditions are key drivers of poor well-being. Without real concern for these, mental health care becomes little more than a cosmetic exercise. Human rights are about more than individual freedoms. Community rights, equality and building community and society must be paramount.

With the above in mind, mental health advocates have called for a social justice approach. This is about engaging 'individuals as coparticipants in decisions which directly affect their lives; it involves taking some action, and educating individuals in order to open possibilities, and to act with value and respect for individuals and their group identities, considering power differentials in all areas of counseling practice and research' (Toporek et al., 2006: 10). The focus therefore moves to the individual-in-their-environment and includes an array of activities by health care providers in the interest of clients and their community, such as empowerment, advocacy and social action. Empowerment has been described as action taken with a client to facilitate their ability to act in the face of oppression, whereas social action is action by the health care professional, external to the client, to confront or act on behalf of client groups.

Another component of mental health care for social justice is raising consciousness of current systemic problems and of available alternatives (Goodman et al., 2004). Such an approach could focus on preventing mental health problems, not only via anti-stigma or awareness programmes, but also by improving socio-economic conditions which lead to problems. As individuals with mental health problems are more likely to experience financial and social hardship arising from their mental health, and those of lower socio-economic status are also more likely to develop mental health problems, one can argue that improving socio-economic circumstances is critical. A report from the UN rapporteur in 2018 revealed how poverty is wide-spread in the UK and leads to mental stress. The report recommended the government take active steps to reduce inequality and raise living standards (UN, 2018). This report is one of many detailing how austerity measures adversely affect the economy, employment, productivity and mental health (e.g. Stiglitz, 2015). One conclusion from this work is that governments should actively seek to empower citizens to gain control over their lives, and develop the external and internal resources to live a meaningful and satisfying life. Some initiatives have been developed, but these projects have remained small-scale and lack funding.

NEOCOLONIALISM

History instructs us that all major civilisations grew by expanding their territories, which meant invading foreign lands, oppressing and enslaving others. Consequently, relationships have often been determined by the difference between dominators and dominated. The socio-economic impact of this power imbalance has often been described, but it was Fanon (1952/1967) who drew attention to the mental health impact of colonial oppression. As discussed in Chapter 2, socio-economically oppressed individuals experience lower self-esteem and stress, lack control in determining their own lives, and are socially segregated. Despite decolonisation, power differences persist, for example sex or economic slavery, and financial and military imbalances between countries. At the time of writing, there are 25 military and political conflicts in the world (Council on Foreign Relations, 2018). There are also large international economic differences, with smaller economies dependent on larger ones and therefore vulnerable to misuse of power and foreign aid (Moyo, 2009).

The export of concepts and systems from western mental health care to non-western countries can be considered neo-colonial (Mills, 2014). A WHO (2001) report declaring that hundreds of millions of people worldwide are suffering at any one time from a mental or brain disorder and that many have no mental health policy with many people not getting the mental health care they need led to the formation of the Movement for Global Mental Health, which strives 'to close the treatment gap for people living with mental disorder worldwide' (Patel et al., 2011: 88), by using a standard approach for all countries and health sectors.

As discussed in Chapter 4, the 'standard approach' the Global Mental Health Movement seeks is premised on the idea that mental health problems are 'illnesses' with underlying biological components. Consequently, the majority of interventions introduced in countries without mental health care focus on pharmaceutical treatment, based on psychiatric diagnoses derived from the DSM or ICD. The biomedicalisation of mental health is at odds with the subjective experiences and illness perceptions that individuals in non-western countries have: 'cultural interpretations are downplayed and regarded secondary to conquering the "scientific" challenge of "mental illness"'; consequently, the global mental health movement 'inadvertently plays into the hands of a different set of interests', usually those of Big Pharma (Thomas et al., 2005: 26). This has engendered the 'McDonaldization of mental health care' and the rapid spread of psychiatric care, while local solutions for mental health problems are dismissed (Timimi, 2010: 686). The attribution of distress to aberrant brain chemistry also diverts attention from social conditions and inequalities that may instigate distress (Parker, 2014a). Biomedical interventions thus create 'pills for life's ills' (Moncrieff, 2009: 105).

In summary, the export of western mental health problems may lead to further neo-colonialisation, and to an exacerbation of mental health problems. The alternative is to stimulate the development of local models and solutions for mental health care, while striving to improve socio-economic inequalities.

THE BRAVE NEW WORLD OF MENTAL HEALTH CARE

Previous sections have discussed how powerlessness, capitalist ideology and weak human rights may have led policy makers to structure mental health care in a way that fails for many. However, one cannot avoid positing a more sinister reason behind current policies. The failure of health care may well have been an intentional aim rather than an unwanted side-effect. The treatments provided to most (drugs and brief CBT) carry the implication that there is something wrong with clients: it personalises and individualises problems. There is little or no money allocated to in-depth approaches that empower individuals and enable them to see the complexity of their problems, including societal problems. The contemporary mental health care system in actuality obstructs empowerment and stands ideologically opposed to demands for socio-economic change with the population steered toward an acceptance of their misery as fate.

People in power have always sought to manipulate the minds of other people. In Roman times emperors sought popularity by dispensing 'bread and circuses' – happiness in the short term in the midst of long-term structural disempowerment. Manipulation strategies are nowadays more refined. At the beginning of the 20th century, Freud's cousin, Bernard Bernays, used psychoanalysis to promote commercial products. He named his discipline 'public relations'. Shortly afterwards, National Socialism took this to a new level. After the Second World War, many philosophers (Hannah Arendt, Erich Fromm and others) wrote about the programmability of human beings, fearing a 'Brave New World' in which people would become programmed willing accomplices of the state, lost in their own private search for pleasure.

The dark history of mental health care is rarely spoken about: the Nazi psychiatrists, drug experiments on inmates, the incarceration of political opponents in Communist Russia – labelled as insane – the use of drugs, electric shock treatment and brainwashing (Marks, S., 2018), and on the other side of the Atlantic, the CIA's development of brainwashing techniques (isolation, hooding, forced standing, and deliberate destruction of existing personal identity). The CIA's handbook for these procedures is still used in Guantanamo Bay (Selisker, 2016). These are notorious examples, but manipulation techniques and micro-control have also been employed in regular mental health hospitals.

Psychotherapy, brainwashing and religious conversion have much in common (Frank & Frank, 1961). Owing to the vulnerability of clients, therapists have power which they could potentially misuse to incrementally change the minds of clients (Ecclestone, 2017). Therapists can consciously or unconsciously mould clients in the direction of what they see as the perfect citizen, making therapy a potential place for coercion (Hinshelwood, 2018). Indeed, in several countries treatment is used to manipulate individuals to conform to wider societal norms (Zhang, 2017). In religious communities also, particularly in the US, LGBTQI individuals can visit a conversion therapist who attempts to remodel them as straight.

The idea that governments might intentionally use mental health care to manipulate a population is plausible. There are numerous examples of how Conservative government ministers intentionally developed policies that have produced known harmful effects (Jones, 2016). In the 1980s, education policy directives led to reduced classes on critical thinking and critical history (Forrester & Garrett, 2016). In more recent years, the Conservatives have been accused by their coalition partner, the Liberal Democrats, of deliberately failing to build social housing, through the fear that this would lead to people voting Labour. Perhaps, most serious of all, the UN rapporteur (UN, 2018) has argued that austerity measures have been deliberately used in the UK for ideological reasons despite the known harm they produce. The NHS Digital's Adult Psychiatric Morbidity Survey (McManus et al., 2016) shows that while more than 43% of benefit claimants have attempted suicide, this vulnerability has been ignored in decision making. The government responded to the UN report with outright denial, refusing to answer questions about the known consequences of its policies. The introduction of a cap on benefits that a family can receive has caused a significant increase in debts, mental health problems and suicide attempts, and again the government refuses to answer questions about this practice (Savage, 2018).

To the above selection of policy initiatives designed to induce harm or restrict the ability of citizens can be added the use of social media in political campaigning to produce shifts in public opinion. These have played a significant and disturbing role in the US presidential election of 2016 and the UK referendum on EU membership. Firms such as Cambridge Analytica have targeted PR campaigns on Facebook to nudge population voting patterns. Politics is placing increasing attention on the psychological manipulation of the population. Indeed, what is called 'psychological governance' is now recognised as central to the operation of contemporary capitalism (Roberts, 2018).

The employment of mass psychological techniques through social media and the use of nudge psychology suggests that future conflicts may be decided not just by what happens on the street. The key battles may not be so much about who controls physical space as who controls psychological space. One of the arguments against the widespread use of psychiatric drugs is that they numb psychological responses to adversity. It cannot be forgotten that awareness of harm wrought in the social arena has long been a driver of social change. Current mental health policy may thus, intentionally or otherwise, have the effect of suppressing demands for necessary social change. This could be considered an essential aspect to an ideological stance that represents ethical and political problems as medical ones. We should therefore be little surprised that government ministers have not recommended that insight-giving therapies be given a higher priority in the mental health toolbag. The aim of mental health care must be about more than making people feel better – or just good enough to prevent rioting.

When we consider much of official mental health policy – the medicalisation of social and political problems, the elevation of happiness as a social and economic good, the exclusion of users' voices from policy debates, the privatisation of services, public health and advertising campaigns to deliver a 'corporate' sanctified view of mental health – we must remain fiercely sceptical of the current unedifying mainstream political construction of mental health.

CULTURAL ANXIETY-MANAGEMENT

Why has the mental health care system been reorganised at this particular moment in Britain's history? What does this say about the wider culture in the UK? Why do people not rebel against the undermining of the NHS? Several psychodynamic and existential authors have posed these questions. The organisational changes, they argue, are created by a specific culture, and this culture is further stimulated by it. This is the culture of anxiety that people attempt to avoid and deny.

People have many realistic reasons to be anxious, as the introductory chapter showed. There are many ways how people can cope with this fear. Existential threats – such as we are now facing – often provoke conservative responses, people narrow their horizons, becoming more nationalistic, focusing on traditional values such as the family, and discriminating against people we do not know. On a political level, we see the re-emergence of strands of political thought and outright fascism that we thought had been left behind in the 1930s. On top of that several countries seek to close their borders and build walls to prevent others entering.

Our culture appears to be one in which we find it difficult to sit with our anxieties and suffering (Davies, 2011). That is, instead of examining where our anxieties originate or learning to live with them, we want a quick solution. Roosevelt famously said that the only thing we have to fear is fear itself, the implication of which is that we learn to face our fears head on. Nowadays, politicians have another tale to tell. They can solve our fears for us – fears which are magnified by projecting them outwards onto specific groups such as immigrants or the EU.

In our era of extreme anxiety and limited anxiety tolerance, the mental health system has been reorganised in such a way that it results less in anxiety reduction in clients and more in anxiety elevation in staff. With mental health care McDonaldised to give rapid on-demand solutions to the patient-customers, short-term satisfaction is the order of the day – existential hunger awaits in the long term (De Wachter, 2012; Kunneman, 2005)! The medicalisation of distress enables health care workers to manage the suffering that they are confronted with, and the medicalisation of misery renders people unable to comprehend their experiences in ordinary, meaningful terms (Rapley et al., 2011).

Public mental health services can be regarded as a psychological defence against overwhelming anxieties (Rizq, 2012a). The government's IAPT programme seems to have resulted in 'a perversion of care where NHS mental health services now disavow the realities of suffering, dependence and vulnerability and turn away from the complexities of managing those in psychological distress' (Rizq, 2012b). Many treatments offered (particularly online self-help or psycho-education material) are solution-focused interventions, which convey the idea that there can be a quick solution for every problem. There is limited time in the therapies to teach service users to sit with their emotions – just feel what you feel, analyse and take time before jumping to conclusions. The consumerist ethos further underlines this idea, that you can choose a tailor-made solution and all your troubles will be gone. The pain and effort of working through emotions, and acknowledging reality as a source of them, gets short shrift in this model. The idea that the complexity of lived experiences can be reduced to a simple set of options is confirmed in the proliferation of surveillance aimed at monitoring and evaluating staff and clinical activity. The obsession with a small range of de-personalised quantitative questionnaires – ignoring the complexity of clients' lived experiences – seems to be a symbolic attempt to gain mastery over feelings that we unconsciously try to avoid.

A specific example of this continuous surveillance is the obsession with managing risk in mental health care (Stanford et al., 2017). One of the first things that a patient encounters when they ask for support is a risk assessment. What is the risk that you will harm yourself or others? Assessors are required to undertake such risk assessments to cover their own legal liability and to justify their actions to their manager. So individuals are not merely regarded as being 'at risk' for experiencing mental health problems, they *are* 'a risk'. This reflects our obsession with risks in neoliberal culture (Beck, 1992). This risk culture has reduced clients to objects of calculation in mental health care, a suicide risk number or a warning note in their file. The risk paradigm affects not only the relationship between service user and service provider, but also the clients' well-being, self-image and stigma (Rizq, 2017).

One of the future focus points of IAPT are online interventions. If present trends continue, practitioners will offer therapy in an imaginary world, divorced from connections in the here-and-now with a real person who can confront the patient. However, individuals need a real other to be able to see their blind spots. Self-help can be beneficial but usually accords with the way we already see ourselves. It is our self-gaze that the gaze of another human being can break through, and that we cannot get from sitting alone in front of a computer. This online virtual world becomes a safe world to which we can flee and where we will not feel discomfort. This is a make-believe world masquerading as reality. A place where simple solutions abound, where we can pretend the problems are not in the real world. With this focus on the virtual and the imaginary, the mental health system becomes the culturally accepted symbol that helps us to avoid reality. It further confirms the avoidance of reality that many already engage in, fleeing to an online second life. To optimise this function of splitting the real from the imaginary, the mental health system is reduced to interventions which prevent confrontation with the real. IAPT in this guise becomes yet another instance of self-governance and obsession with the self.

This culture of anxiety management should be taken seriously, and attention given (in policy making, public debate, education and therapy) to learning how to tolerate uncertainty and anxiety. The emphasis on risk management in therapeutic settings should be critically analysed and transformed, so that a more constructive relationship can emerge which enables clients to thrive and the therapist to be unafraid of what could go wrong. In this way vulnerability can be used as a tool for change.

10

EDUCATIONAL CRISIS

Joel Vos

THE POLITISATION OF EDUCATION

Neutral education does not exist. Perhaps the most obvious illustration of this concerns how ethnic conflicts are presented to school children in conflict areas (Peled-Elhanan, 2012). The vast majority of maps in Israeli and Palestinian schoolbooks somehow 'forget' to present the existence of the other entity, leading to children growing up with 'an internal representation of their homeland, in which one does not include the other' (Adwan et al., 2014). Only 4% of maps in Palestinian textbooks and 24% of Israeli books show differences between Palestinian areas and Israel, and present all territorial names. When officials in the Israeli department of education proposed including maps with the UN borders in school books, they faced professional repercussions and votes of no-confidence in parliament. The impact of this politisation of the school curriculum is far-reaching, with research showing that young people of one group see themselves as the only victim and the other group as the sole aggressor. This black-or-white teaching polarises and exacerbates the conflict. We see in cases such as this that political ideologies manifest themselves via the education curriculum and teaching style, and manipulate children's perceptions of the world, their subjectivity and their being-in-the-world (Freire, 1970/2018). This chapter describes how politicians influence the education and well-being of children and young people in the UK and other countries, and what alternatives are available to this.

YOUNG MINDS FOR SALE

Foucault teaches us not only that neutral education doesn't exist but that it cannot. Value-free facts are impossible (Ball, 2012). We cannot escape the influence of the dominant ideology in a society. In different eras, different aspects of our experiences and our world are opened up to light whilst others are cast into darkness and forgotten (Thomson, 2001). Educated to avoid them, we remain unaware of these blind spots. We therefore tend to accommodate new information without undermining the fundamental ideas we already subscribe to. Since the 1980s, governmental policies have prescribed the curriculum for state schools. This social control function of schooling offers a 'hidden curriculum' that is non-academic and implicit, but significant for the well-being of pupils, their teachers, family and future society (Vallance, 1973).

Education has always been political, and successive governments have attempted to impose reforms to shape the curriculum (Forrester & Garratt, 2016). The national education system was founded in the UK at the end of the 19th century, with elementary education purposefully kept at a low level with a rudimentary curriculum focused on reading, writing and arithmetic. The authoritarian teaching style encouraged docility, and obedience in both pupils and teachers. Initiative was discouraged in order to circumvent working-class children questioning their socio-economic position. After World War Two, free secondary education was added. This resulted in the tripartite system of grammar, secondary modern and technical schools, with pupils allocated to a school according to their ability, assessed by the 11-plus exam. With differences in parental support, in teaching and class-specific items present in the tests, the result was socio-economic differentiation: working-class children were likely to be referred to schools where they learned skills for manual labour and middle-class children to schools preparing them for white-collar jobs.

Until the 1970s, teachers had relative freedom over curriculum content and pedagogical methods. This came under fire after the publication of *The Black Papers*, a series of publications condemning child-centred progressive education. In 1976, the 'great debate' was ignited by Prime Minister James Callaghan, who blamed progressive teachers for inadequate skills and knowledge. He argued for education to be primarily focused on socio-economic aims. Callaghan desired learning to be structured in the form of a 'core curriculum' of basic knowledge and vocational skills, to prepare pupils for the workplace. The Office for Standards in Education (Ofsted) was established to monitor and ensure that schools delivered this curriculum. At the end of the 1980s, this was followed by the introduction of Standard Assessment Tasks (SATs) to determine children's ability. Simultaneously, financial control over schools was devolved, with headmasters managing budgets and competing with other schools for parents' favour in league tables.

Consequently, teachers became trapped between the twin pillars of accountability and the duty to follow a coerced curriculum. For schools to be evaluated as good, teachers had to deliver a lean curriculum and restricted teaching style focused on basic knowledge that would lead to good SATs scores. It was argued that this system gave teachers greater freedom, but in practice teachers had more to do and less time to do it, with larger classes, less individual attention, and less space given over to social well-being, mental health, critical thinking and creativity. The narrow focus on testing, a standard curriculum, skills-based teaching and memorisation skills emphasised a conformist pedagogy marked by a vulgar instrumentality. Aronowitz & Giroux (1986/2003: 24) provide a dismal summary of the resulting educational 'Bleak House':

> instead of helping students to think about who they are and what they should do … teachers have been trained to use techniques, control student discipline, teach a given subject effectively and organise a day's activities as efficiently as possible.

The lack of 'discretionary time' for teaching mental, social and critical skills is not coincidental. The education minister Keith Joseph exhibited his disdain for developing social, psychological and critical thinking skills in the 1983 White Paper 'Teaching Quality' (Wright & Bottery, 2002). He undermined initiatives toward these and insisted on personally approving subject teaching syllabuses to ensure the vocational goal-directedness of the curriculum (Wilkin, 1996).

As education policies undermined the possibility of learning critical thinking skills and side-lined any prospect of building community, what is at stake is not just the ability to be creative but the capacity for conceptual thought itself. This development weakens the foundations of democracy, as awareness, self-reflection and critical thinking are necessary for active participation in society (Aronowitz & Giroux, 1986/2003). For Arendt (1970: 417), the capacity for critical reflection was key to understanding failures of democracy. In her view it was not stupidity but a curious 'inability to think' that underpinned the popularity of the National Socialists. That 'neoliberal violence in education' now 'wages a war' against the critical skills of 'questioning the givens, in philosophy as well as politics and art' (Castoriadis, 1997) should fill us with foreboding.

In the eyes of its critics, the governments of New Labour and the 2010 Tory-Liberal coalition gave conservative and neoliberal values in the organisation of the education system 'meat and teeth' (Exley & Ball, 2011: 110). The neoliberal agenda was endorsed in a flurry of white papers on 'Education for Citizenship' in the early years of the Blair government, while similar debates on citizenship took place in other European countries. In the UK the debate centred on teaching 'fixed British core values' – a toxic presupposition which rejected different opinions and expected minorities to adjust. The prescription of these 'values' can be seen as opening salvoes in a discursive war to mould citizenship to accept Britishness and nationalism as conflated concepts. The central value in this newly constructed Britishness seemed to be self-sustenance, a concept ill at ease with the founding principles of the welfare state. Instead of teaching social and life skills and reinforcing the sense of a common community, individuals were now to be responsible for themselves – success or failure being reframed in individual and moral terms.

In this environment, lack of interest and motivation on the part of learners is attributed to their own shortcomings. Whereas past governments may have provided support for citizens, individuals must now govern themselves (Foucault, 2012). This has produced a public intolerance of failure, with newspapers pointing the finger at 'lazy scoundrels' living on benefits. The outcome of the Brexit referendum is one consequence of this discourse of self-sustenance and British pride. A further one is that individuals are expected to be a success, even though the system provides insufficient support for developing skills in social and mental domains. Failure is now deemed the upshot of either immorality or craziness. By having teachers promulgate these values, pupils learn to govern themselves – an inexpensive form of auto-policing.

Thus, the structure of the school system now embodies neoliberal values, such as efficiency, cost-effectiveness, self-sustenance and competition. Classrooms are structured to 'reproduce capitalist relations of production', reflecting and preparing pupils for their future position in the market place (Althusser, 2014). The know-how that the industry needs is reflected in the curriculum, and the social relations in the classroom reflect future workplace hierarchies. So too, the culture of disciplined learning, docility and oppression, lack of democratic voting, and the punishment of oppositional behaviour reflects the wider work culture (Bourdieu &

Passeron, 1990). Social structures in schools normalise inequality and injustice, and inhibit critical-oppositional behaviour. Furthermore, the Confederation of British Industry (CBI) has described how individuals are now responsible and accountable for developing their own qualifications and skills. 'Lifelong learning' in reality shifts responsibility from employers to employees: workers must adjust to job demands, not vice versa.

Research suggests that young minds are not only moulded by the hidden curriculum at school but also by the hidden programming in the media and gaming industry. Governments and corporations have long used films, advertisements and shows to create stereotypes and popularise ideas (Shaw & Youngblood, 2010). In recent decades, powers have turned to the Internet, social media and games. The entertainment industry popularises themes such as urban conflict and warfare, using stereotypes of physically charged males portraying toxic forms of masculinity as normal. These forms are now invading official public recruitment films for the armed forces, aided and abetted by movies and programmes depicting the country under relentless attack from foreign powers. This subliminally stimulates a continuous emotional state of threat and nationalism. Numerous studies have been conducted on the political and psychological effects of such violent representations with a plethora of contradictory conclusions. There is evidence that research findings can be bought, with some authors having ties with the gaming industry or Hollywood (Johnson et al., 2013). Despite the lack of scientific consensus, it is unquestionable that attitudes and perceptions of people are influenced and that young people are particularly vulnerable to manipulation and addiction (Kuss & Griffiths, 2012).

MENTAL HEALTH IMPACT

The neoliberal turn in education described above has undoubtedly influenced the mental health of young people. First, by influencing the lifestyles and values of pupils by reinforcing capitalist values. The repeated emphasis on educational and professional success creates a narrow sense of meaning in life. It is not surprising that later in life career is prioritised over leisure time, family and community – anything which points to a greater purpose in life beyond money. This paucity of support for social and existential-spiritual meanings in life may induce a lower sense of fulfilment and poorer psychological well-being (Vos, 2018).

Second, children develop a technical rationality about life. The focus of education on positivism (e.g. universal laws and empirical testability) occludes the sacred, rituals and social assemblies. In their wake comes disenchantment, social disconnection and self-orientedness. The championing of technical rationality can shut out any appetite for the subjective, including emotional life. It imprints the functionalistic idea that everything in life can be achieved and controlled, if one tries hard enough. This illusion of controllability renders individuals vulnerable to chronic frustration, existential anxiety and personal failure.

Third, individuals who struggle to progress on the educational-professional ladder may develop a sense of meaninglessness and low self-esteem. Instead of blaming the system, the education system teaches that they are responsible for their failure. Consequently, when someone cannot find appropriate work and needs state support, they are treated as failures, deemed in need of cognitive therapy.

Fourth, education reforms have led to increased pressures for teachers, with concomitant stress and burnout. Larger class sizes make it impossible for teachers to give sufficient attention to everyone. As a result, they lack the time and skills to improve group dynamics when a child shows disruptive behaviour. Again, the consequence is that the child's behaviour and not the systemic source of any difficulty becomes problematised. Children with disruptive behaviour are at increased risk of being pathologised and seen as needing individual counselling or pharmaceutical treatment. This disadvantages children from backgrounds with low socio-economic status or family problems.

Fifth, there is clear evidence that labelling children and young people can lead to stigmatisation and social exclusion, affecting their sense of self, participation in the community and well-being (Pescosolido et al., 2007). Because of this, critics have called for normalisation and inclusive education. There have been many pioneers in inclusive education, but the reality is that many teachers lack the skills and resources, and children end up excluded. Fortunately, successful projects of inclusive education do exist, but these seem limited to specific cases in some countries (Rix et al., 2005).

MENTAL HEALTH CARE

We are in the midst of an epidemic of 'psychiatric disorders' in young people. Never before have so many been given psychiatric labels such as ADHD and Autism. In the UK, between 2% and 12.5% of individuals between 5 and 18 years have been diagnosed, and annually 42,000 are hospitalised because of self-harm

(Green et al., 2005). Young people nowadays experience more emotional problems than three decades ago (Collishaw et al., 2004). This has been attributed to a complex interaction of factors, including individual child characteristics, family, school, socio-economic circumstances and society (Midgley et al., 2017).

Overall, mental health care has moderately positive effects on young people's well-being – many indicate they have benefitted from therapy (Hanley & Noble, 2017). It is also relatively cost-effective. It is estimated that the cost of a mental health problem over childhood is almost 22 times the average cost of therapy (Place2B, 2010). However, the UK invests relatively little in children's health care, and it has been suggested that less than half of those who need or want help receive it (Knapp et al., 2016). Differences exist in the efficacy of types of treatment for different individuals. A range of treatments is proven, including humanistic, psychodynamic, play and CBT. Treatments focusing on the child within their social context (e.g. family therapy) seem particularly effective (Roth & Fonagy, 2006).

Psychiatric drugs are increasingly prescribed to young people, something which reflects the neoliberal context more than actual needs and recovery rates (Timimi, 2010). Research shows that such drugs can permanently alter brain structures (Andersen, 2005). A thorny issue in medicalisation is the lack of consent, as young people do not commonly self-refer, may not understand the implications of treatment, and may be unable to resist professional coercion.

Finally, UK national health care guidelines recommend stepped-care for children and adolescent mental health care. There is no systematic research supporting this. More positive findings exist for initiatives that move away from this by orienting the care system around the needs and goals of children and young people (Timimi, 2013).

EDUCATIONAL ALTERNATIVES

This chapter has shown how young people's minds may be manipulated for political ends, and how this adversely affects mental health. Solutions have been proposed. These focus on the dynamics present in the peer group, the family and the wider community of the child, raising social-political awareness, developing critical thinking skills, encouraging reflection on fundamental values for life, confronting difficult topics and being realistic about the complexities of life. These approaches are well supported by evidence (Creemers & Kyriakides, 2007). Below, several successful projects are outlined.

Pupils, teachers and schools benefit from projects to improve understanding of mental health (Weare & Nind, 2011). The Life Skills-Based Education Programme, launched by the WHO in 1999, targeted the psychosocial competences of children and young people, such as critical and creative thinking, decision making and problem solving, communication, relationships, self-awareness, empathy, and coping with emotions. Researchers have shown that projects are particularly beneficial when they start at an early age, use a whole-school approach for longer than a year, and engender a sustainable change in a school's ethos. It is helpful to focus on the promotion of mental health rather than prevention of mental illness: to train teachers, to liaise with parents and educate them, and involve the wider community. Supporting children and young people in the development of their identity, by accepting and stimulating their involvement in youth subcultures, finds support in research which shows that social ties, a sense of belonging and peer acceptance are important.

There are several early interventions which can help to prevent antisocial behaviour (Rix et al., 2005). Addressing behaviour from the perspective of group dynamics and social roles can be effective in de-escalating problems. These approaches do not imply that disruptive behaviour is tolerated or that mental health problems are minimised, but rather that the problem is identified and multiple perspectives are brought to bear to cope with it.

Many school-wide philosophies about holistic and humanistic schooling have also been developed. The Steiner model encourages unity of mind, body and soul, free from state shackles and the imposition of a core curriculum (Childs, 1991). Several schools follow a democratic philosophy, lifting discipline and instead focusing on children's interests and their emotional life. These follow the principles advocated by John Dewey (1923). The Summerhill School in the UK offers weekly meetings where children discuss mutually agreed codes and to cope with breaches (Forrester & Garratt, 2016).

Many teachers have based their education on critical pedagogy (Freire, 1970/2018). This sees education as a collaborative process between teachers and pupils. Before study can attain significance for a pupil, the teacher may need to show them the significance of the study for their life. Freire promoted critical thinking skills in students, particularly the ability to decode the social and political meanings of texts (Aronowitz & Giroux, 1986/2003). Pupils are stimulated to develop an understanding of their social context, and how this influences them, for example by debating cultural diversity, which doesn't necessarily take 'British core values' as given, but explores the historical and social context of colonialism, migration, labour shortages in industrialised countries and so on. This process of conscientisation moves beyond theoretical reflexivity, and explores actions that individuals can engage in. From the perspective of critical pedagogy, the best way to stimulate mental health is to challenge society's myths, to perceive more clearly its reality and limitations, and to formulate alternatives.

Many of the above-mentioned solutions are included in the Finnish education model dubbed the 'miracle of education' (Niemi et al., 2016). In Finland, the school system is largely decentralised, with no inspectors or national tests. It is based on a culture of trust in the teachers' and headmasters' professionalism. There is a core curriculum, but schools have freedom to develop their own programme. There are several cross-curricular themes such as personal growth, cultural identity and internationalism, media skills and communication, participatory citizenship and entrepreneurship, responsibility for the environment, well-being and a sustainable future, safety and traffic, and technology. Education begins at the age of 7 and the school hours are amongst the lowest in the western world. Any student with learning or adjustment problems receives a personal learning plan, and can receive remedial teaching in or alongside regular classroom education or else can be transferred to special needs education which, when feasible, is inclusive. This system appears successful. Finnish pupils rank highest in many international league tables in literacy skills. They also experience some of the highest levels of well-being and happiness in the world (Määttä & Uusiautti, 2012).

The success of the Finnish model demonstrates that radical change of the education system is possible, that such transformation is feasible in a short timeframe and that this can produce better mental health and stronger communities. We have two options, according to Freire (1970/2018): education as a practice of freedom or as an instrument to facilitate integration into the status quo.

11

VISIONS FOR MENTAL HEALTH CARE

Joel Vos

> We cannot dismantle one system, without having another in its place.
>
> Ghandi, 1973

Visionaries of radical change have always been the victim of disbelief, but this has not stopped them from struggling for a better world. Although Bevan was told it was impossible to establish a free national health service, the UK recently celebrated the 70th anniversary of the NHS. Its history offers hope that structural change can be achieved quickly. This chapter offers some guides for better mental health care, to tackle the crises described in previous chapters. We envisage a society in which individuals and communities experience agency, security, connection, meaning and trust, and in which governments stimulate these key indicators.

CONTEXT-ORIENTED CARE

Many chapters have shown how mental health problems are not only caused by individual factors such as biology, childhood trauma or unhelpful coping skills. Mental health is influenced by social context. However, traditional care and one-size-fits-all approaches such as IAPT often focus on individual factors. We advocate a model that focuses on delivering the type of care that a specific person needs at a specific moment within a specific domain of their life (see Figure 11.1 and Table 11.1).

There needs to be systematic assessment of how different domains give rise to distress. This could be formally recorded alongside the distress via psychosocial ICD/DSM codes (Allsopp & Kinderman, 2017). Instead of personalising problems, wider social circles should first be addressed. As Van Deurzen (2009: 131) writes, 'People are defined by their relation to a physical world, to other people, to themselves and to their network of meaning.'

The *global domain* includes wider crises which directly or indirectly impact people, for example socio-economic inequality, climate crisis and politics. Governments could protect human rights and reduce inequality, not only via international laws but through active policies to enhance people's lives.

The *societal domain* includes nationwide situations which affect people, such as stigma, housing problems, racism, unemployment and the benefits system. Mental health care at societal level includes education provision which teaches critical thinking and life skills, prevention campaigns, a fair benefits system and a just legal system.

In the *community*, individuals can experience problems in the neighbourhood, work conditions, relationships with friends, colleagues and others or in certain social activities. Mental health care could involve interventions at all these levels. Physically improving neighbourhoods, community building activities, providing just social housing, social work, mediation, couples and family therapy and open dialogues are just a few examples.

The *daily life domain* comprises the immediate experiences of an individual in interaction with the wider world, and may include stresses at work and home, lifestyle, coping skills, environmental mastery, and sense of self-efficacy. Mental health care could include support for the interaction between the individual and their context, for example training in life-skills, social-skills, employment-skills or lifestyle.

The *emotional domain* is the traditional focus of mental health care. This includes individual experiences, as well as self-esteem, chronic stress and common psychological concerns. Troubling emotions can be caused by unresolved concerns in the wider social domains, and similarly these emotional concerns have the potential to create wider problems. A variety of mental health care options should therefore be available to match the unique needs of the individual.

Biology is the domain of medicine, which includes the psychological impact of chronic or life-threatening diseases, where medical care can provide relief, for example via medical treatments for pain control. It is possible that some individuals may have a biological predisposition to psychiatric problems, and if support at other social domains has not resolved anything, psychiatric or psychopharmaceutical care may be considered.

The domain of *existential-spiritual self* is implicitly present in all domains; this concerns the sense of being author of your own life, and how you fundamentally relate to surrounding social domains, with a sense of freedom and responsibility within the boundaries of your social contexts. This includes the sense of larger meaning, purpose or spirituality in life.

A starting point to explore the social domains can be to encourage clients to tell their stories and discover patterns and regularities in the expression and experience of distress. This replaces the question 'What is wrong with you?' with four others: 'What has happened to you?' (How has Power operated in your life?); 'How did it affect you?' (What kind of Threats does this pose?); 'What sense did you make of it?' (What is the meaning of these situations and experiences to you?); 'What did you have to do to survive?' (What kinds of threat response are you using?). These questions describe coping and survival mechanisms which may functional in conflicts and adversities in both past and present. This approach follows the power-threat-meaning framework as an alternative to DSM/ICD-diagnoses (Johnstone et al., 2018).

This approach helps clients regain personal agency within the constraints of social contexts. Within each domain, the aim of care should be to help individuals see and use their capacity for change, while accepting the reality of limitations. This could imply that individuals develop external resources, such as applying for financial support, to improve their housing and may also include advice such as hiking, going into nature or visiting museums, which doctors in some countries (e.g. Scotland) already prescribe. Individuals could also develop internal resources such as communication, coping or emotional skills.

Which domain should be addressed depends on an individual's stories and their consciousness of their social context. Conscientisation is the process through which individuals develop awareness of how their socio-cultural context influences their life, and their own role in this. Critical education has an important role in this process, and community activities and daily life skills training can help. If individuals see a therapist, they should be supported in critically analysing the social context of their problems, and becoming conscious of what is meaningful for them within a given context (Vos, 2018).

Finally, therapists must be cognisant of the mind-manipulating trends in society and mental health care. As described in other chapters, the mind is now a key strategic site in capitalist society. Psychological therapies, however, can be used as a counterforce. Watts (2017) has argued that psychotherapy can help people 'resist the brainwashing of armies, bureaucracies, churches and corporations'.

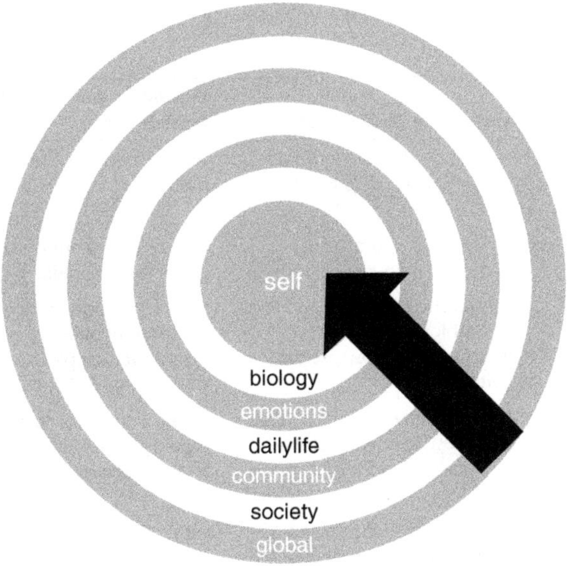

Figure 11.1 Mental health in context: life domains (arrow represents the directions of steps in mental health care beginning with global intervention)

Via continuous reflexivity, personal therapy and supervision, therapists can become aware of how power imbalances enter the therapy room.

POLICY MAKERS AND ORGANISATION STRUCTURE

We recommend a fundamental rethinking of the mental health system in the light of social justice as human rights with a primary focus on empowerment to live a meaningful and satisfying life. This implies a variety of approaches matched and tailored to individuals-in-their-social-context. Seen from a social justice perspective, mental health care should be delivered by professionals who provide an authentic, understanding relationship. Within this framework people can be helped to become conscious of their social context and develop the freedom and agency to flourish in it. This implies challenging discrimination, developing culturally sensitive treatments, offering a variety of treatments, and overcoming conflict and obstacles to participation in society.

The current system for determining funding and policy making suggests that vested interests operate. To improve the situation policy makers should

Table 11.1 Overview of domains with examples for individuals and mental health care

domain	Example for individuals	Examples for mental health care
global	climate crisis, socio-economic inequality, sense of justice/injustice	reduce inequality, human rights protection, policies
society	stigma, housing problems, racism, unemployment, benefits	education, parenting support, prevention, benefits system, law
community	neighbourhood, work conditions, relationships with friends, colleagues and others, social activities	neighbourhood improvement, community building, social work, mediation, couples and family therapy, open dialogue
daily life	daily stress at work and home, lifestyle, coping skills, environmental mastery, self-efficacy	life skills training, social skills training, employment training, lifestyle advice, dietician
emotions	self-esteem, chronic stress and common psychological concerns	variety of psychological care options
biology	chronic or life-threatening physical diseases, genetics, endogenic psychiatric problems	physical care, psychiatry, psychopharmaceuticals
self	author of their own life; fundamental sense of self; relationships to domains; sense of freedom and responsibility	existential or spiritual care

include a representative sample of stakeholders, with real power for each member. Economists should have a non-determining role in final decision making. The content of the service should be the primary aim of the service, not the balance sheet with service users involved in the strategic and policy decision making at all levels. Mental health advocates could play a larger role in mental health care, reaching beyond their current remit on individual care (Newbigging et al., 2015).

To prevent corruption, there must be full transparency over budgets, policy-making processes, and potential conflicts of interests. Reviews of care quality should be conducted by independent experts, be double-checked by other relevant authorities, and include a wide variety of evaluation data, including the subjective voices of service users and staff. Furthermore, funding should be allocated via a neutral general pot of money where proposals are selected on merit. Current allocation is skewed toward psychiatric drugs and CBT.

SPECIFIC EXAMPLES

Housing first

Individuals with severe persistent mental health problems often live in low-quality housing that is physically inadequate, crowded, noisy and located in undesirable neighbourhoods. They are more likely to feel excluded from community activities (Boardman et al., 2010). Many people with mental health problems are homeless. Traditional programmes focus primarily on improving the psychological problems of homeless individuals. However, in many countries the Housing First campaigns start with improving housing circumstances, which has shown to help individuals better, quicker and cheaper (Aubry et al., 2015).

Open Dialogue

Successful approaches tapping into the social resources of individuals have recently emerged. Open Dialogue, Avoin Vuoropuhelu, a Finnish need-adapted approach to psychosis that stresses flexibility, rapid response to crisis, family-centred therapy meetings, and individual therapy. It focuses on social networks by encouraging dialogues between the treatment team, the individual and the wider social network. Research suggests that open dialogues reduce duration of psychosis, and lead to functional recovery with minimal use of drugs (Lakeman, 2014).

PASS

Since 2000, there have been numerous projects in European countries to improve access to mental health care. Permanent Access to Mental Health Care, Permanent Accès aux Soins de Santé (PASS) in France comprises hospital-based multidisciplinary units providing primary care services to patients who lack health care coverage. They use a whole-person approach, combining health and social care. Research indicates that PASS makes it easier for individuals in socially disadvantaged situations to access care, and care that is directed at multiple domains of the individual's life (Georges-Tarragano, 2015).

Reconciliatory community projects

War and ethnic conflicts can lead to widespread mistrust, anxieties and hardened attitudes. Political conflicts can lead to a vicious cycle, as those targeted develop traumatic symptoms such as hyper-vigilance and black-and-white thinking.

To break this cycle, individuals need to have a safe space for healing. There are many initiatives to help reconciliation (Rosoux & Anstey, 2017). Specific community projects and sensitive counselling exist to heal inter-generational and ongoing trauma in indigenous people whose land has been stolen and who endure structural discrimination (Mitchell, 2016). Reconciliation is complex and requires a delicate balancing act between the interests of different parties. A lesson from previous peace and reconciliation efforts is that simultaneous interventions in multiple social domains are necessary.

Existential approaches

A wide range of practitioners give explicit attention to existential and humanistic topics. Research shows that many clients benefit from these (Elliott et al., 2013), particularly when there is a focus on helping individuals to live a meaningful and satisfying life despite problems. Compared with other care approaches, existential therapies and counselling appear effective in improving the psychological well-being of individuals in liminal life situations (Vos, 2016, 2018). Most existential therapies share a holistic-humanistic approach, where the social context including that of the therapeutic relationship is explicitly considered (Van Deurzen & Arnold-Baker, 2018). Existential practitioners use relational, existential, experiential, phenomenological, mindfulness and meaning-oriented skills – all evidence-based.

Participatory action research

Traditional research merely describes or observes individuals but action research deliberately attempts to improve the well-being of individuals and communities. This means that all stakeholders participate in crucial phases of research, with input into the development and evaluation of workshops or other experiments in social improvement. Many projects have helped individuals in marginalised communities (Kemmis & McTaggart, 2005).

Lobbyists

Numerous charities, professional bodies and mental health care advocate lobbying for better mental health care (see Table 11.2). Several books have been written about mental health lobby strategies (Drebing, 2016), creating social change and using direct action (Engler & Engler, 2016). For example,

Table 11.2 Selection of large mental health charities and lobbyists

United Kingdom	United States
BACP British Association for Counselling and Psychotherapy	AAGC American Academy of Grief Counseling
BAAT Black African and Asian Therapy Network	ACA American Counseling Association
BPC British Psychological Society	Active Minds
Care in Mind	AFSP American Foundation for Suicide Prevention
Critical Psychiatry Network	AGPA American Group Psychotherapy Association
Critical Psychotherapy Network	AMHCA American Mental Health Counselors Association
COSCA Counselling and Psychotherapists in Scotland	APA American Psychological Association
Cruse Bereavement Care	ASCA American School Counseling Association
DPAC Disabled People Against Cuts	Child Mind Institute
Drive	ICPN International Critical Psychiatry Network
Free Psychotherapy Network	Mad in America
Hearing Voices Network	MHA Mental Health America
Institute Voices Network	NAADAC National Association for Alcoholism and Drugs Abuse Counselors
Life Skills Foundation	NAMI National Alliance on Mental Health Illness
Mental Health Foundation	NIHM National Institute for Mental Health
Mental Health Resistance Network	Stonewall
Mental Health UK	Trans Lifeline
Metal for Life	Treatment Advocacy Center
Migrant's Right Network	
Mind	
MQ Mental Health	
National Counselling Society	
NSUN National Survivor User Network	
Pink Therapy	
Psychologists for Social Change (prior: Psychologists Against Austerity)	
Punk4MentalHealth	
Rethink	
Samaritans (phone support line)	
Sane	
SEAP Advocacy. Support Empower Advocate Promote	
Survivors' Trust	
Together	
UKCP UK Council for Psychotherapy	
UKAHPP UK Association for Humanistic Psychology Practitioners	
Young Minds	

Psychologists for Social Change use several tactics: engaging in systems thinking (seeing problems and solutions as part of the system); mobilising/training the profession; sharing knowledge (public campaigns, political lobbying);

working directly with service users; using community psychology; aiming for empowerment and equality of vulnerable groups; and developing constructive relationships between service provider and service user drawing on knowledge, abilities and resources of both.

Economic lobbyists have argued that mental health care is a cost-efficient way of reducing mental health problems and cutting its negative annual impact of £70–£100 billion on the economy almost in half, such as reducing welfare benefits, sickness days, lost productivity at work and crime. Community care is particularly cost-effective (e.g. by reducing expensive in-patient admissions). Similarly, skills training, education and prevention campaigns increase well-being at population level at low costs (Jané-Llopis et al., 2005). With an effectiveness of less than 10%, the money spent on 90% of the patients in IAPT could be invested in more effective care, such as tailored humanistic/relational or existential/spiritual care. Psychopharmaceutical drugs usually do not enhance structural recovery from problems and lead to long-term dependency on pills, and are therefore relatively cost-inefficient; consequently, using pills only as last resort can lead to long-term savings. Finally, economists have argued that economic growth not only requires individuals being free from severe mental health problems, but that they also have the right skills to contribute creatively and effectively (Wahlbeck, 2015). This necessitates a holistic mental health care system that offers empowerment, skills, education and positive opportunities. It is this system that we envisage as the solution to the crises in mental health.

REFERENCES

Aboraya, A., Rankin, E., France, C., El Missiry, E., & John, C. (2006). The reliability of psychiatric diagnosis revisited. *Psychiatry, 3*(1): 41–50.

Adams, A. E., Sullivan, C. M., Bybee, D., & Greeson, M. R. (2008). Development of the scale of economic abuse. *Violence Against Women, 14*(5), 563–588.

Adams, T. V. (2016). *The psychopath factory: how capitalism organises empathy.* London: Repeater Books.

Adwan, S., Bar-Tal, D., & Wexler, B. E. (2014). Victims of our own narratives? Portrayal of the 'other' in Israeli and Palestinian school books. *Political Psychology, 37*(2).

Afifi, M. (2007). Gender differences in mental health. *Singapore Medical Journal, 48*(5), 385.

Allen, J., Balfour, R., Bell, R., & Marmot, M. (2014). Social determinants of mental health. *International Review of Psychiatry, 26*(4), 392–407.

Allen, K., Mendick, H., Harvey, L., & Ahmad, A. (2015). Welfare Queens, thrifty housewives, and do-it-all mums: celebrity motherhood and the cultural politics of austerity. *Feminist Media Studies, 15*(6), 907–925.

Allsopp, K., & Kinderman, P. (2017). A proposal to introduce formal recording of psychosocial adversities associated with mental health using ICD-10 codes. *The Lancet Psychiatry, 4*(9), 664–665.

Althusser, L. (2014). *On the reproduction of capitalism.* London: Verso.

American Psychiatric Association (APA) (1980). *Diagnostic and statistical manual of mental disorders* (3rd ed.). Washington, DC: American Psychiatric Association.

American Psychiatric Association (APA) (2010). *American Psychiatric Association practice guideline for the treatment of patients with major depressive disorder* (3rd ed.). Available at https://psychiatryonline.org/pb/assets/raw/sitewide/practice_guidelines/guidelines/mdd.pdf (accessed June 2018).

American Psychiatric Association (APA) (2013). *Diagnostic and statistical manual of mental disorders* (5th ed.). Arlington, VA: American Psychiatric Association.

Andersen, S. L. (2005). Stimulants and the developing brain. *Trends in pharmacological sciences, 26*(5), 237–243.

Andresen, R., Oades, L. G., & Caputi, P. (2011). *Psychological recovery: beyond Mental illness.* Chicester: Wiley.

Angermeyer, M., & Matschinger, H. (2005). Causal beliefs and attitudes to people with schizophrenia: trend analysis based on data from two population surveys in Germany. *British Journal of Psychiatry, 186,* 331–334.

Arendt, H. (1970). Thinking and moral considerations: a lecture. *Social Research, 38/3,* Fall.

Arendt, H. (1978). *The life of the mind. Book two: Willing*. London: Harvest.

Aronowitz, S., & Giroux, H. A. (1986/2003). *Education under siege*. London: Routledge.

Aubry, T., Nelson, G., & Tsemberis, S. (2015). Housing first for people with severe mental illness who are homeless: a review of the research and findings from the at home – chez soi demonstration project. *The Canadian Journal of Psychiatry, 60*(11), 467–474.

Back, L. (2016). *Academic diary*. London: Goldsmiths Press.

Baker, S. (2011). Dean criticised by tribunal is promoted. *Times Higher Education*, 28 July. Available at www.timeshighereducation.com/news/dean-criticised-by-tribunal-is-promoted/416955.article?sectioncode=26&storycode=416955&c=1 (accessed July 2015).

Ball, S. (2012). *Foucault, power, and education*. London: Routledge.

Bank, D., & Buckman, R. (2002). Gates Foundation buys stakes in drug makers. *Wall Street Journal*, 17 May.

Barkham, M., & Saxon, D. (2018). The effectiveness of high-intensity CBT and counselling alone and following low-intensity CBT: a reanalysis of the 2nd UK National Audit of Psychological Therapies data. *BMC Psychiatry, 18*(1), 321.

Baumberg, B. (2016). The stigma of claiming benefits: a quantitative study. *Journal of Social Policy, 45*(2), 181–199.

BBC News Online (2008). University staff faking survey. 13 May. Available at http://news.bbc.co.uk/1/hi/education/7397979.stm (accessed June 2017).

BBC News Online (2011). After scandal, what happens now to University of Wales? Available at www.bbc.co.uk/news/uk-wales-15463655 (accessed July 2017).

BBC News Online (2015). Economy tracker: unemployment. Available at www.bbc.co.uk/news/10604117 (accessed November 2018).

Beck, U. (1992). *Risk society: towards a new modernity*. London: Sage.

Becker, G. (1992). The economic way of looking at life. Nobel lecture. Available at https://www.nobelprize.org/uploads/2018/06/becker-lecture.pdf (accessed December 2018).

Bentall, R. (2012). *Doctoring the mind: why psychiatric treatments fail*. London: Penguin.

Beresford, P., Nettle, M., & Perring, R. (2010). *Towards a social model of madness and distress? Exploring what service users say*. London: Joseph Rowntree Foundation.

Berry, J. W., & Kim, U. (1988). Acculturation and mental health. In P. R. Dasen, J. W. Berry, & N. Sartorius (Eds.), *Cross-cultural research and methodology series, Vol. 10. Health and cross-cultural psychology: toward applications* (pp. 207–236). Thousand Oaks: Sage.

Bhugra, D. (2004). Migration and mental health. *Acta Psychiatrica Scandinavica, 109*(4), 243–258.

Bhugra, D. (2006). Severe mental illness across cultures. *Acta Psychiatrica Scandinavica, 113*(Suppl. 429), 17–23.

Binnie, J. (2015). Do you want therapy with that? A critical account of working within IAPT. *Mental Health Review Journal, 20*(2), 79–83.

Boardman, J., Killaspy, H., & Mezey, G. (Eds.). (2010). *Social inclusion and mental health*. London: Royal College of Psychiatrists.

Boseley, S. (2018). The drugs do work: antidepressants are effective, study shows. *Guardian*, 21 February.

Bourdieu, P., & Passeron, J. C. (1990). *Reproduction in education, society and culture.* London: Sage.

Boym, S. (2001). *The future of nostalgia.* New York. Basic Books.

Boym, S. (2010). *Another freedom: the alternative history of an idea.* London: University of Chicago Press.

Boym, S. (2017). *The off-modern.* London: Bloomsbury.

Bracken, P., Thomas, P., Timimi, S., & Asen, E. (2012). Psychiatry beyond the current paradigm. *British Journal of Psychiatry, 201*(6), 430–434.

British Medical Association (BMA) (2018). Lost in transit: funding for mental health services in England. Available at www.bma.org.uk/collective-voice/policy-and-research/public-and-population-health/mental-health/funding-mental-health-services (accessed December 2018).

Broom, D. H., D'Souza, R. M., Strazdins, L., Butterworth, P., Parslow, R., & Rodgers, B. (2006). The lesser evil: bad jobs or unemployment? A survey of mid-aged Australians, *Social Science and Medicine, 63*(3), 575–586.

Brown, M. (2017). Antidepressants work, so why do we shame people for taking them? *Guardian*, 1 September.

Busby, E. (2018). Universities make 'misleading' marketing claims to students, report suggests. *Independent*, 21 September.

Campbell, E. G., Weissman J. S., Ehringhaus S., Rao, S. R., Moy, B., Feibelmann, S., & Goold, S. D. (2007). Institutional academic–industry relationships. *JAMA, 298*(15), 1779–178.

Cantwell, S., Rae, J., Vos, J., & Cooper, M. (2015). How do therapists pose questions to clients about therapeutic methods? BPS Division of Counselling Psychology Annual Conference.

Carlat, D. (2010). *Unhinged: the trouble with psychiatry.* London: Free Press.

Carney, C., McNeish, S., & McColl, J. (2005). The impact of part-time employment on students' health and academic performance: a Scottish perspective. *Journal of Further and Higher Education, 29*(4), 307–319.

Castoriadis, C. (1997). Democracy as procedure and democracy as regime. *Constellations, 4*(1), 1–18.

Chakrabortty, A. (2018). Mis-sold, expensive and overhyped: why our universities are a con. *Guardian*, 20 September.

Children's Commissioner (2017). *Briefing: children's mental health care in England.* Available at www.childrenscommissioner.gov.uk/wp-content/uploads/2017/10/Childrens-Commissioner-for-England-Mental-Health-Briefing-1.1.pdf#page=6 (accessed December 2018).

Childs, G. (1991). *Steiner education in theory and practice.* Edinburgh: Floris Books.

Chomsky, N. (1967). The responsibility of intellectuals. *New York Review of Books, 8*(3), Supp.

Chomsky, N. (2011). *The state-corporate complex: a threat to freedom and survival.* Lecture, University of Toronto, 7 April.

Cimpean, D., & Drake, R. E. (2011). Treating co-morbid chronic medical conditions and anxiety/depression. *Epidemiology and Psychiatric Sciences, 20*(2), 141–150.

Cipriani, A., Furukawa, T.A., Salanti, G., Chaimani, A., Atkinson, L.Z., Ogawa, Y., et al. (2018). Comparative efficacy and acceptability of 21 antidepressant drugs for the acute treatment of adults with major depressive disorder: a systematic review and meta-analysis. *The Lancet, 391*, 10128, 1357–1366.

Clark, D. M. (2018). Realizing the mass public benefit of evidence-based psychological therapies: the IAPT program. *Annual Review of Clinical Psychology, 14*, 159–183.

Clements, J., & Davies, E. (2013). Prevention of psychosis: creating societies where more people flourish. In J. Read and J. Dillon (Eds.), *Models of madness: psychological, social and biological approaches to psychosis* (2nd ed.) (pp. 295–304). London: Routledge.

Clery, E., Curtice, J. & Harding, R. (2017). *British Social Attitudes: the 34th Report*. London. NatCen Social Research, Available online at: www.bsa.natcen.ac.uk

Collishaw, S., Maughan, B., Goodman, R., & Pickles, A. (2004). Time trends in adolescent mental health. *Journal of Child Psychology and Psychiatry, 45*(8), 1350–1362.

Constantine, M. G., Myers, L. J., Kindaichi, M., & Moore III, J. L. (2004). Exploring indigenous mental health practices: the roles of healers and helpers in promoting well-being in people of color. *Counseling and Values, 48*(2), 110–125.

Cooke, R., Barkham, M., Audin, K., Bradley, M., & Davy, J. (2004). Student debt and its relation to student mental health. *Journal of Further and Higher Education, 28*(1), 53–66.

Cooper, J. E., Kendell, R. E., Gurland, B. J., Sharpe, L., Copeland M. R., and Simon R. J. (1972). *Psychiatric diagnosis in New York and London*: Maudsley Monograph No 20. London: Oxford University Press.

Cosgrove, L., Krimsky, S., Vijayaraghavan, M., & Schneider, L. (2006). Financial ties between DSM-IV panel members and the pharmaceutical industry. *Psychotherapy and Psychosomatics, 75*(3), 154–60.

Cotton, E. (2017). The future of therapy. Available at http://eprints.mdx.ac.uk/23197/1/The%20Future%20of%20Therapy%20eBook.pdf (accessed December 2018).

Council on Foreign Relations (2018). Home page. Available at www.cfr.org (accessed November 2018).

Cox, J. L. (2018). *Transcultural psychiatry*. London: Routledge.

Creemers, B., & Kyriakides, L. (2007). *The dynamics of educational effectiveness: a contribution to policy, practice and theory in contemporary schools*. London: Routledge.

Crocker, J., & Major, B. (1994). Reactions to stigma: the moderating role of justifications. In J. M. Olson, & M. P. Zanna (Eds.), *The psychology of prejudice: the Ontario symposium* (pp. 289–314). Hillsdale, NJ: Lawrence Erlbaum.

Davies, J. (2011). Positive and negative models of suffering: an anthropology of our shifting cultural consciousness of emotional discontent. *Anthropology of Consciousness, 22*(2), 188–208.

Davies, J. (2013). *Cracked: why psychiatry is doing more harm than good*. London: Icon Books.

Davies, J. (Ed.). (2017). *The sedated society: the causes and harms of our psychiatric drug epidemic*. London: Palgrave Macmillan.

Davies, J., & Read, J. (2018). A systematic review into the incidence, severity and duration of antidepressant withdrawal effects: are guidelines evidence-based? *Addictive Behaviors*, 4 September. Available at https://doi.org/10.1016/j.addbeh.2018.08.027 (accessed January 2019).

Davies, W., (2015). *The happiness industry: how the government and big business sold us well-being*. London: Verso.

De Almeida, J. C., Frasquilho, D., Zózimo, J., & Parkonnen, J. (2018). EU compass for action on mental health and well-being. Annual Report 2018. Available at https://ec.europa.eu/health/sites/health/files/mental_health/docs/2018_compass_activityreportsummary_en.pdf (accessed December 2018).

De Haan, A. M., Boon, A. E., de Jong, J. T., & Vermeiren, R. R. (2018). A review of mental health treatment dropout by ethnic minority youth. *Transcultural Psychiatry*, *55*(1), 3–30.

De Wachter, D. (2012). *Borderline times: het einde van de normaliteit [the end of normality]*. Tielt: Lannoo Meulenhoff.

De Witte, H., Pienaar, J., & De Cuyper, N. (2016). Review of 30 years of longitudinal studies on the association between job insecurity and health and well-being: is there causal evidence? *Australian Psychologist*, *51*(1), 18–31.

Deleuze, G., & Guattari, F. (2004). *Anti-Oedipus: capitalism and schizophrenia*. Minneapolis, MN: University of Minnesota Press.

Department of Health and Social Care (DHSC) (2018). Hansard: prescriptions drugs – written question – 128871. Available at www.parliament.uk/business/publications/written-questions-answers-statements/written-question/Commons/2018-02-21/128871/ (accessed July 2018).

Devlin, H., & Marsh, S. (2018). Hundreds of academics at top UK universities accused of bullying. *Guardian*, 28 September.

Dewey, J. (1923). *Democracy and education: an introduction to the philosophy of education*. London: Macmillan.

Dick, P. K. (2014). *Lie, Inc.* London: Gollancz.

Dong, D., & Temple, B. (2011). Oppression: a concept analysis and implications for nurses and nursing. *Nursing Forum*, *46*(3), 169–176.

Drebing, C. (2016). *A practical guide to recovery-oriented practice: tools for transforming mental health care*. Oxford. Oxford University Press.

Duvall Smith, A. (2006). Thousands of students 'join sex trade to fund degrees'. *Independent*, 31 October.

Ecclestone, K. (2017). Behaviour change policy agendas for 'vulnerable' subjectivities: the dangers of therapeutic governance and its new entrepreneurs. *Journal of Education Policy*, *32*(1), 48–62.

Ecclestone, K., & Hayes, D. (2009). *The dangerous rise of therapeutic education: how teaching is becoming therapy*. London: Routledge.

Ecks, S. (2005). Pharmaceutical citizenship: antidepressant marketing and the promise of demarginalization of India. *Anthropology and Medicine*, *12*(3): 239–254.

Economou, M., Peppou, L. E., Louki, E., & Stefanis, C. N. (2012). Medical students' beliefs and attitudes towards schizophrenia before and after undergraduate psychiatric training in Greece. *Psychiatry Clin. Neurosci.*, *66*(1):17–25.

Ehrenreich, B. (2010). *Smile or die. How positive thinking fooled America and the world.* London: Granta.

El-Gingihy, Y. (2018). *How to dismantle the NHS in 10 easy steps.* Winchester: Zero Books.

Elliott, R., Greenberg, L. S., Watson, J. C., Timulak, L., & Freire, E. (2013). Research on humanistic-experiential psychotherapies. In M. J. Lambert (Ed.), *Bergin & Garfield's handbook of psychotherapy and behavior change* (6th ed.) (pp. 495–538). New York. Wiley.

Engler, M., & Engler, P. (2016). *This is an uprising: how nonviolent revolt is shaping the twenty-first century.* New York. Nation Books.

Equality and Human Rights Commission (2017). Distributional results for the impact of tax and welfare reforms between 2010–17, modelled in the 2021/22 tax year. Available at www.equalityhumanrights.com/sites/default/files/impact-of-tax-and-welfare-reforms-2010-2017-interim-report_0.pdf (accessed January 2019).

Equality Trust (2018). Submission to the UN Special Rapporteur regarding the linkages between poverty and the realization of human rights in the United Kingdom. Available at www.equalitytrust.org.uk/equality-trust-submission-un-special-rapporteur (accessed December 2018).

Erickson-Schroth, L., & Carmel, T. C. (2016). Transgender mental health. *Psychiatric Annals, 46*(6), 330–331.

European University Association (2007). *Lisbon declaration: Europe's universities beyond 2010.* Brussels: European University Association.

Evans, G. W., Wells, N. M., & Moch, A. (2003). Housing and mental health: a review of the evidence and a methodological and conceptual critique. *Journal of Social Issues, 59*(3), 475–500.

Evans, M. (2004). *Killing thinking: the death of the university.* London: Continuum.

Exley, S., & Ball, S. J. (2011). Something old, something new ... understanding Conservative education policy. *The Conservative Party and Social Policy*, 97–118.

Fanon, F. (1952/1967). *Black skin, white masks* (transl. Markmann, C. L.). New York: Grove Press.

Faulkner, N., & Dhati, S. (2017). *Creeping fascism: Brexit, Trump and the rise of the far right.* London: Public Reading Rooms.

Fazackerley, A. (2018). 2VCs on ... will Brexit damage UK universities? *Guardian*, 20 September.

Fernando, S. (2010). *Mental health, race and culture* (3rd ed.). Houndmills: Palgrave Macmillan.

Fisher, M. (2009). *Capitalist realism: is there no alternative?* Winchester: Zero Books.

Fletcher, D. R., & Wright, S. (2018). A hand up or a slap down? Criminalising benefit claimants in Britain via strategies of surveillance, sanctions and deterrence. *Critical Social Policy, 38*(2), 323–344.

Ford, M. (2015). *The rise of the robots: technology and the threat of mass unemployment.* London: Oneworld.

Forder, J., Jones, K., Glendinning, C., Caiels, J., Welch, E., Baxter, K., Davidson, J., Windle, K., Irvine, A., King, D., & Dolan, P. (2012). Evaluation of the personal health budget pilot programme. Discussion paper, Department of Health.

Forrester, G., & Garratt, D. (2016). *Education policy unravelled.* London: Bloomsbury.

Foucault, M. (2002). *The birth of the clinic.* London: Routledge.

Foucault, M. (2003). *Madness and civilization*. London: Routledge.

Foucault, M. (2012). *Discipline and punish: the birth of the prison*. London: Vintage.

Frances, A. (2012). DSM-5 field trials discredit APA. Available at www.psychologytoday.com/us/blog/dsm5-in-distress/201210/dsm-5-field-trials-discredit-apa (accessed December 2018).

Frances, A. (2013). *Saving normal*. New York: William, Morrow.

Frank, J. D., & Frank, J. B. (1961). *Persuasion and healing: a comprehensive study of psychotherapy*. Baltimore, MD: Johns Hopkins University.

Fredrickson, B. L., & Roberts, T. A. (1997). Objectification theory: toward understanding women's lived experiences and mental health risks. *Psychology of Women Quarterly*, *21*(2), 173–206.

Freedman, R., Lewis, D. A., Michaels, R., Pine, D. S., Schultz, S. K., Tammings, C. A., Gabbard, G. O., Gau, S. S., Javitt, D. C., Oquendo, M. A., Shrout, P. E., Vieta, E., & Vieta, E., & Yager, J. (2013). The initial field trials of DSM-5: new blooms and old thorns. *American Journal of Psychiatry*, *170*, 1–5.

Freire, P. (1970/2018). *Pedagogy of the oppressed*. London: Penguin.

Fromm, E. (1941/2011). *Escape from freedom*. New York: Ishi Press.

Fromm, E. (1973). *The crisis of psychoanalysis*. Harmondsworth: Penguin.

Fukuyama, F. (1992). *The end of history and the last man*. London: Penguin.

FullFact (2018). Mental Health. https://fullfact.org/health/mental-health-there-are-fewer-beds-nurses-and-psychiatry-trainees-2010/ (accessed December 2018).

Furedi, F. (2011). Introduction to the marketisation of higher education and the student as consumer. In M. Molesworth, R. Scullion, & E. Nixon (Eds.), *The marketisation of teaching and learning in higher education* (pp. 1–7). New York. Routledge.

Furedi, F. (2016). *What's happened to the university?* London: Routledge.

Georges-Tarragano, C. (2015). Les permanences d'accès aux soins de santé (PASS): tradition d'hospitalité et modèle d'organisation innovante. *La Revue de Médecine Interne*, *36*(1), 38–41.

Gibbs, A. (2018). Anti-depressants do work – but children need someone to talk to. *Observer*, 4 March.

Gilburt, H. (2016). Trust finances raise concerns about the future of the Mental Health Taskforce recommendations. *King's Fund Blog*, *14*.

Gillies, V. F., & Edwards, R. (2017). 'What about the children?' Re-engineering citizens of the future. In J. Pykett, R. Jones, & M. Whitehead (Eds.), *Psychological governance and public policy* (pp. 96–115). London: Routledge.

Glasby, J., & Tew, J. (2015). *Mental health policy and practice*. London: Palgrave Macmillan.

Goodman, L. A., Liang, B., Helms, J. E., Latta, R. E., Sparks, E., & Weintraub, S. R. (2004). Training counseling psychologists as social justice agents: feminist and multicultural principles in action. *The Counseling Psychologist*, *32*(6), 793–836.

Gostin, L. O., & Gable, L. (2004). The human rights of persons with mental disabilities: a global perspective on the application of human rights principles to mental health. *Maryland Law Review*, *63*, 20.

Gøtzsche, P. (2013). *Deadly medicines and organised crime: how big pharma has corrupted health care*. London: Radcliff.

Grant, J. M., Mottet, L. A., Tanis, J., Herman, J. L., Harrison, J., & Keisling, M. (2010). *National transgender discrimination survey report on health and health care*. Washington, DC: National Center for Transgender Equality and the National Gay and Lesbian Task Force.

Green, F., Felstead, A., & Burchell, B. (2000). Job insecurity and the difficulty of regaining employment: an empirical study of unemployment expectations. *Oxford Bulletin of Economics and Statistics, 62*, 855–883.

Green, H., McGinnity, Á., Meltzer, H., Ford, T., & Goodman, R. (2005). *Mental health of children and young people in Great Britain, 2004*. Houndmills: Palgrave Macmillan.

Greenslit, N. (2005). Depression and consumption. *Culture, Medicine and Psychiatry, 29*, 477–501.

Grey, N., Byrne, S., Taylor, T., Shmueli, A., Troupp, C., Stratton, P., Sefi, A., Law, R., & Cooper, M. (2018). Goal-oriented practice across therapies. In M. Cooper, & D. Law (Eds.), *Working with goals in psychotherapy and counselling* (pp. 181–203). New York. Oxford University Press.

Griffin, P. (2015). Crisis, austerity and gendered governance: a feminist perspective. *Feminist Review, 109*(1), 49–72.

Guardian (2018a). Letters: Why we are sceptical of anti-depressant analysis. *Guardian*, 23 February.

Guardian (2018b). Letters: Anti-depressants work – and we are the proof. *Guardian*, 1 March.

Hanley, T., & Noble, J. (2017). Therapy outcomes: is child therapy effective? In N. Midgley, J. Hayes, & M. Cooper (Eds.), *Essential research findings in child and adolescent counselling and psychotherapy*. London: Sage.

Happé, F., & Ronald, A. (2008). The 'fractionable autism triad': a review of evidence from behavioural, genetic, cognitive and neural research. *Neuropsychology Review, 18*(4), 287–304.

Harré, R. (2002). *Cognitive science: a philosophical introduction*. London: Sage.

Harrell, S. P. (2000). A multidimensional conceptualization of racism-related stress: implications for the well-being of people of color. *American Journal of Orthopsychiatry, 70*(1), 42–57.

Harrington, A. (2012). The body's role in human experience. *Fora TV*. Available at http://fora.tv/2012/03/24/Being_Human_Individual__Society__Morals__Culture (accessed February 2014).

Harrow, M., Jobe, T. H., & Faull, R. N. (2012). Do all schizophrenia patients need antipsychotic treatment continuously throughout their lifetime? A 20-year longitudinal study. *Psychol. Med., 42*(10), 2145–2155.

Health Foundation (2018). *A place to grow*. Available at http://reader.health.org.uk/a-place-to-grow (accessed January 2019).

Healy, D. (2006). Did regulators fail over selective serotonin reuptake inhibitors? *British Medical Journal, 333*(7558), 92–95.

Hengartner, M. P., Angst, J., & Rössler, W. (2018). Antidepressant use prospectively relates to a poorer long-term outcome of depression: results from a prospective community cohort study over 30 years. *Psychotherapy and Psychosomatics, 87*, 181–183.

Herman, E. S., & Chomsky, N. (1994). *Manufacturing consent: the political economy of the mass media*. London: Vintage.

Herman, J. L. (1992) Trauma and Recovery. New York. Basic Books.

Hieronymus, F., Lisinksi, A., Nilsson, S., & Eriksson, E. (2017). Efficacy of selective serotonin reuptake inhibitors in the absence of side effects: a mega-analysis of citalopram and paroxetine in adult depression. *Molecular Psychiatry*, 25th July. DOI 10.1038/mp.2017.147. Available at www.nature.com/mp/journal/vaop/ncurrent/full/mp2017147a.html?foxtrotcallback=true (accessed September 2017).

Hinshaw, M. (2007). *The mark of shame: stigma of mental illness and agenda for change*. Oxford: Oxford University Press.

Hinshelwood, R. D. (2018). *Therapy or coercion: does psychoanalysis differ from brainwashing?* London: Routledge.

Hodges, L. (2009a). Scandal of the students who never sat exams. *Independent*, 26 November.

Hodges, L. (2009b). Trouble at the top: Malcolm Gillies' departure from City University has revealed an intense relationship between governors and vice-chancellors. *Independent*, 12 August.

Huxley, A. (1932). *Brave New World*. London: Chatto & Windus.

Hwang, S. W. (2001). Homelessness and health. *Canadian Medical Association Journal, 164*(2), 229–233.

Imison, C., Naylor, C., Buck, D., Curry, N., Addicott, R., & Zollinger-Read, P. (2011). *Transforming our healthcare system*. London: The King's Fund.

Independent Office for Police Conduct (IOPC) (2018). New research reveals major barriers for people with mental health concerns making a complaint about policing. Available at www.policeconduct.gov.uk/news/new-research-reveals-major-barriers-people-mental-health-concerns-making-complaint-about (accessed January 2019).

Insel, T. (2013). Transforming diagnosis. Available at www.nimh.nih.gov/about/director/2013/transforming-diagnosis.shtml (accessed February 2014).

Institute for Public Policy Research (IPPR) (2017). Not by degrees: improving student mental health in the UK's universities. Available at www.ippr.org/files/2017-09/1504645674_not-by-degrees-170905.pdf (accessed October 2018).

Institute of Fiscal Studies (2017). Higher education funding in England: past present and options for the future. IFS Briefing Note BN211. Available at www.ifs.org.uk/uploads/publications/bns/BN211.pdf (accessed July 2017).

International Lesbian, Gay, Bisexual, Trans and Intersex Association's (ILGA) (2018). State-sponsored homophobia report. Available at https://ilga.org/state-sponsored-homophobia-report (accessed December 2018).

Jablensky, A., Sartorious, N., Emberg, G., Anker, M., Korten, A., Cooper, J. E., Dar, R. & Bertelsen, A. (1992). Schizophrenia: manifestations, incidence and course in different cultures: a World Health Organisation 10-country study. *Psychological Medicine*, Suppl. *20*, 1–97.

Jacobson, L. H., & Cryan, J. F. (2007). Feeling strained? Influence of genetic background on depression-related behavior in mice: a review. *Behavior Genetics, 37*(1), 171–213.

Jané-Llopis, E., Barry, M., Hosman, C., & Patel, V. (2005). Mental health promotion works: a review. *Promotion & Education, 12*(2_suppl), 9–25.

Johnson, D., Jones, C., Scholes, L., & Carras, M. C. (2013). Videogames and wellbeing: a comprehensive review. Melbourne: Young and Well Cooperative Research Centre.

Johnstone, L., & Boyle, M., with Cromby, J., Dillon, J., Harper, D., Kinderman, P., Longden, E., Pilgrim, D., & Read, J. (2018). *The power threat meaning framework: towards the identification of patterns in emotional distress, unusual experiences and troubled or troubling behaviour, as an alternative to functional psychiatric diagnosis.* Leicester: British Psychological Society.

Jones, O. (2016). *The establishment: and how they get away with it.* London: Melville House.

Jorm, A. F., Patten, S. B., Brugha, T. S., & Mojtabai, R. (2017). Has increased provision of treatment reduced the prevalence of common mental disorders? Review of the evidence from four countries. *World Psychiatry, 16*(1), 90–99.

Joseph Rowntree Foundation (2014). Reducing poverty in the UK: a collection of evidence reviews. Available at www.jrf.org.uk/report/reducing-poverty-uk-collection-evidence-reviews (accessed December 2018).

Kagan, C., Burton, M., Duckett, P., Lawthom, R., & Siddiquee, A. (2011). *Critical community psychology.* Chichester: Wiley.

Kagan, J. (2012). *Psychology's ghosts.* New Haven, CT: Yale University Press.

Kalia, A. (2018). Young, gifted – and ready to tackle the mental illness epidemic. *Guardian,* 28 September.

Kelly, G. A. (1955). *The psychology of personal constructs. Vol. 1: A theory of personality.* New York: Norton.

Kelso, P. (2018). 40 people died in 'barbaric' secure hospitals the government pledged would close. *Sky News,* 15 November.

Kemmis, S., & McTaggart, R. (2005) Participatory action research: communicative action and the public sphere. In N. Denzin, & Y. Lincoln (Eds.), *The Sage Handbook of Qualitative Research* (pp. 559–603). Thousand Oaks, CA: Sage.

Kendrick, T. (2015). Long-term antidepressant treatment: time for a review? *Prescriber, 26*(19), 7–8.

Kieselbach, T. (2003). Long-term unemployment among young people: the risk of social exclusion. *American Journal of Community Psychology, 32*(1–2), 69–76.

Kinderman, P. (2014). *A new prescription for psychiatry: why we need a whole new approach to mental health and wellbeing.* London: Palgrave Macmillan.

King's Fund (2018). *Does the NHS need more money and how could we pay for it?* London: King's Fund.

Kitanaka, J. (2013). *Depression in Japan: psychiatric cures for a society in distress.* Princeton, NJ: Princeton University Press.

Klein, N. (2007). *The shock doctrine.* London: Penguin.

Kleinman, A. (1997). Social Suffering. Berkeley, CA: University of California Press.

Kleinman, A. (2012). Rebalancing academic psychiatry: why it needs to happen – and soon. *British Journal of Psychiatry, 201,* 421–422.

Knapp, M., Ardino, V., Brimblecombe, N., Evans-Lacko, S., Lemmi, V., King, D., Snell, T., Murguia, S., Mbeah-Bankas, H., Crane, S., Harris, A., Fowler, D., Hodgekins, J., & Wilson, J. (2016). *Youth mental health: new economic evidence.* London: Personal Social Services Research Unit.

Knifton, L., Gervais, M., Newbigging, K., Mirza, N., Quinn, N., Wilson, N., & Hunkins-Hutchison, E. (2010). Community conversation: addressing mental health stigma with ethnic minority communities. *Social Psychiatry and Psychiatric Epidemiology, 45*(4), 497–504.

Kondro, W., & Sibbald, B. (2004). Drug company experts advised to withhold data about SSRI use in children. *Canadian Medical Association Journal, 170*, 783.

Kunneman, H. (2005). *Voorbij het dikke-ik: bouwstenen voor een kritisch humanisme* [Beyond the fat ego: building blocks for a critical humanism]. Amsterdam: Humanistics University Press.

Kuss, D. J., & Griffiths, M. D. (2012). Internet gaming addiction: a systematic review of empirical research. *International Journal of Mental Health and Addiction, 10*(2), 278–296.

Laing, R. D. (1990). *The politics of experience and the bird of paradise.* London: Penguin.

Lakeman, R. (2014). The Finnish open dialogue approach to crisis intervention in psychosis: a review. *Psychotherapy in Australia, 20*(3), 28.

Lambert, M. J. (Ed.) (2013). *Bergin and Garfield's handbook of psychotherapy and behavior change*. New York. Wiley.

Lantz, S. (2004). Sex work and study: the new demands facing young people and their implications for health and well being. *Traffic*, 3.

Lasalvia, A., Soppei, S., Van Bortel, T., Bonetto, C., Cristofalo, D., Wahlbeck, K., Bacle, S. V., + 11 others (2013). Global pattern of experienced and anticipated discrimination reported by people with major depressive disorder: a cross-sectional survey. *The Lancet, 381*(9860), 55–62.

Lawlor, C., Sharma, B., Khondoker, M., Peters, E., Kuipers, E., & Johns, L. (2017). Service user satisfaction with cognitive behavioural therapy for psychosis: associations with therapy outcomes and perceptions of the therapist. *British Journal of Clinical Psychology, 56*(1), 84–102.

Lawton-Smith, S., Dawson, J., & Burns, T. (2008). Community treatment orders are not a good thing. *The British Journal of Psychiatry, 193*(2), 96–100.

Layard, R. (2006). *The depression report: a new deal for depression and anxiety disorders.* London: Centre for Economic Performance, LSE.

Learning Disabilities Mortality Review (LeDeR) (2017). Annual report. December 2017. Available at www.hqip.org.uk/wp-content/uploads/2018/05/LeDeR-annual-report-2016-2017-Final-6.pdf (accessed December 2018).

Ledford, H. (2013). Psychiatry framework seeks to reform diagnostic doctrine. *Nature*, 12972.

Lennon, M. C., & Rosenfield, S. (1992). Women and mental health: the interaction of job and family conditions. *Journal of Health and Social Behavior*, 316–327.

Lenton, P. (2015). Determining student satisfaction: an economic analysis of the National Student Survey. *Economics of Education Review, 47*, 118–125.

Lerner, M. (2006). *The left hand of God: Taking back our country from the religious right.* Harper Collins.

Levin, D. M. E. (1987). *Pathologies of the modern self: Postmodern studies on narcissism, schizophrenia, and depression.* New York University Press.

Lexchin, J., Bero, L. A., Djulbegovic, B., & Clark, O. (2003). Pharmaceutical industry sponsorship and research outcome and quality: systematic review. *British Medical Journal, 326*, 1167–70.

Li, Z., Page, A., Martin, G., & Taylor, R. (2011). Attributable risk of psychiatric and socio-economic factors for suicide from individual-level, population-based studies: a systematic review. *Social Science & Medicine, 72*(4), 608–616.

Littlewood, R. (2001). *Pathologies of the West: the anthropology of mental illness in Europe and America*. Ithica, NY: Cornell University Press.

Littlewood, R., & Lipsedge, M. (1997). *Aliens and alienists: ethnic minorities and psychiatry* (3rd ed.). London: Routledge.

Liu, J., Hong, M., Yan-Ling, H., Bin X., & 14 others (2011). Mental health system reform in China: history, recent service reform and future challenges. *World Psychiatry, 10*, 210–216.

Lobban, F., Barrowclough, C., & Jones, S. (2005). Assessing cognitive representations of mental health problems. I: The illness perception questionnaire for schizophrenia. *British Journal of Clinical Psychology, 44*(2), 147–162.

Lok, A., Bockting, C. L. H., Koeter, M. W. J., Snieder, H., Assies, J., Mocking, R. J. T., Vinkers, C. H., Kahn, R. S., Boks, M. P., & Schene, A. H. (2013). Interaction between the MTHFR C677T polymorphism and traumatic childhood events predicts depression. *Translational Psychiatry, 3*(7), e288.

Longden, E. (2013). *Learning from the voices in my head*. TED.com: TED Books.

Longden, E., Read, J., & Dillon, J. (2017). Assessing the impact and effectiveness of hearing voices network self-help groups. *Community Mental Health, 54*(2), 184–188.

Lucy-Costlett, R. (2018). Why treating your depression is like learning your times tables. *Guardian*, 28 February.

Lustig, S. L. (Ed.). (2012). *Advocacy strategies for health and mental health professionals: from patients to policies*. New York: Springer.

Määttä, K., & Uusiautti, S. (2012). How do the Finnish family policy and early education system support the well-being, happiness, and success of families and children? *Early Child Development and Care, 182*(3–4), 291–298.

MacDonald, R., Shildrick, T., & Furlong, A. (2014). 'Benefits Street' and the myth of workless communities. *Sociological Research Online, 19*(3), 1–6.

MacLeavy, J. (2011). A 'new politics' of austerity, workfare and gender? The UK coalition government's welfare reform proposals. *Cambridge Journal of Regions, Economy and Society, 4*(3), 355–367.

Maldonado, J. R., & Spiegel, D. (2008). Dissociative disorders: dissociative identity disorder (multiple personality disorder). In R. E. Hales, Yudofsky, S. C., & Roberts, L. W. (Eds.), *The American Psychiatric Publishing textbook of psychiatry* (5th ed.) (pp. 681–710). Washington, DC: American Psychiatric Publishing.

Marcuse, H. (1964). *One dimensional man*. London. Penguin.

Marks, D. F. (2018). IAPT under the microscope. *Journal of Health Psychology, 23*(9), 1131–1135.

Marks, S. (2018). Suggestion, persuasion and work: psychotherapies in communist Europe. *European Journal of Psychotherapy & Counselling, 20*(1), 10–24.

Martin, E. (2009). *Bipolar expeditions: mania and depression in American culture*. Princeton, NJ: Princeton University Press.

Maslej, M. M., Boklker, B. M., Russell, M. J., Eaton, K., Durisko, Z., Hollon, S. D., Swanson, G. M., Thomson, J. A. Jr., Mulsant, B. H., & Andrews, P. W. (2017). The mortality and myocardial effects of antidepressants are moderated by preexisting cardiovascular disease: a meta-analysis. *Psychotherapy and Psychosomatics, 86*, 268–282.

Mason, P. (2015). *Postcapitalism: a guide to our future.* London: Allen Lane.

Matheson, S. L., Shepherd, A.M., Laurens, K.R. & Carr, V.J. (2011). A systematic meta-review grading the evidence for non-genetic risk factors and putative antecedents of schizophrenia. *Schizophrenia Research, 133*(1–3), 133–42.

Mazzucato, M. (2018). *The value of everything: making and taking in the global economy.* London: Allen Lane.

McDaid, D., & Knapp, M. (2010). Black-skies planning? Prioritising mental health services in times of austerity. *The British Journal of Psychiatry, 196*(6), 423–424.

McGrath, L., Griffin, V., & Mundy, E. (2015). *The psychological impact of austerity.* Available at https://psychagainstausterity.files.wordpress.com/2015/03/paa-briefing-paper.pdf (accessed December 2018).

McManus, S., Bebbington, P., Jenkins, R., & Brugha, T. (Eds.) (2016). *Mental health and wellbeing in England: Adult Psychiatric Morbidity Survey 2014.* Leeds: NHS Digital.

Mehta, J., Clifford, C., Taggart, D., & Speed, E. (2018). *Where your mental health just disappears overnight: disabled people's experiences of the employment and support allowance work related activity group. Inclusion.* London: Three Guineas Trust.

Mehta, S. (1997). Is being 'sick' really better? Effect of the disease view of mental disorder on stigma. *Journal of Social and Clinical Psychology, 16*(4), 405–419.

Meyer, B., Pilkonis, P. A., Krupnick, J. L., Egan, M. K., Simmens, S. J., & Sotsky, S. M. (2002). Treatment expectancies, patient alliance, and outcome: further analyses from the National Institute of Mental Health Treatment of Depression Collaborative Research Program. *Journal of Consulting and Clinical Psychology, 70*(4), 1051–1055.

Midgley, N., Hayes, J., & Cooper, M. (Eds.) (2017). *Essential research findings in child and adolescent counselling and psychotherapy.* London: Sage.

Mills, C. (2014). *Decolonizing global mental health: the psychiatrization of the majority world.* London: Routledge.

Mills, C. (2018). Dead people don't claim: a psychopolitical autopsy of UK austerity suicides. *Critical Social Policy, 38*(2), 302–322.

Mitchell, T. (2016). Colonial trauma and political pathways to healing. In S. L. Stewart, R. Moodley, & A. Hyatt (Eds.), *Indigenous cultures and mental health counselling: four directions for integration with counselling psychology* (pp. 141). New York: Routledge.

Moncrieff, J. (2003). *Is psychiatry for sale? an examination of the influence of the pharmaceutical industry on academic and practical psychiatry.* London: King's College, Institute of Psychiatry.

Moncrieff, J. (2009). *The myth of the chemical cure.* Houndmills: Palgrave Macmillan.

Mosher, L. R. (1998). Letter of resignation from the American Psychiatric Association. Available at www.critpsynet.freeuk.com/Mosher.htm (accessed January 2019).

Moyn, S. (2018). *Not enough. Human rights in an unequal world.* Cambridge, MA: Harvard University Press.

Moyo, D. (2009). *Dead aid: why aid is not working and how there is a better way for Africa.* Houndmills: Palgrave Macmillan.

National Committee of Inquiry into Higher Education (1997). *Higher education in the learning society: main report.* London: HMSO. Available at www.educationengland.org.uk/documents/dearing1997/dearing1997.html (accessed January 2019). https://bei.leeds.ac.uk/Partners/NCIHE/ (accessed March 2009).

Negt, P., Brakemeier, E. L., Michalak, J., Winter, L., Bleich, S., & Kahl, K. G. (2016). The treatment of chronic depression with cognitive behavioral analysis system of psychotherapy: a systematic review and meta-analysis of randomized-controlled clinical trials. *Brain and Behavior, 6*(8), e00486.

Newbigging, K., Ridley, J., McKeown, M., Sadd, J., Machin, K., Cruse, K., De La Haye, S., Able, L., & Poursanidou, K. (2015). *Independent mental health advocacy – the right to be heard: context, values and good practice.* London: Jessica Kingsley.

Newcomb, M. E., & Mustanski, B. (2010). Internalized homophobia and internalizing mental health problems: a meta-analytic review. *Clinical Psychology Review, 30*(8), 1019–1029.

NHS (National Health Services UK) (2017). *Health Survey for England.* London. NHS.

NHS Digital (2017). Prescriptions dispensed in the community: Statistics for England, 2007–2016. Available at https://digital.nhs.uk/data-and-information/publications/statistical/prescriptions-dispensed-in-the-community/prescriptions-dispensed-in-the-community-england---2007---2017 (accessed July 2018).

NICE (2009) *Depression. The treatment and management of depression in adults (NICE guideline).* National Institute for Health and Clinical Excellence. www.nice.org.uk

Niemi, H., Toom, A., & Kallioniemi, A. (Eds.) (2016). *Miracle of education: the principles and practices of teaching and learning in Finnish schools.* New York. Springer.

O'Brien, M., & Kyprianou, P. (2017). *Just managing? What it means for the families of austerity Britain.* Cambridge: Open Book.

Office for National Statistics (2018). Estimating suicide among higher education students, England and Wales: experimental statistics. Available at www.ons.gov.uk/releases/estimatingsuicideamonghighereducationstudentsenglandandwales (accessed October 2018).

Orford, J. (2008). *Community psychology: challenges, controversies and emerging consensus.* Chichester: Wiley.

Orlowski, J. P., & Wateska, L. (1992). The effects of pharmaceutical firm enticements on physician prescribing patterns. *Chest, 102,* 270–273.

Orwell, G. (1949). *1984.* London: Secker & Warburg.

Paris, J. (2013). *Fads and fallacies in psychiatry* (p. 5). London: Royal College of Psychiatrists.

Parker, I. (2014a). *Psychology after deconstruction* (pp. 68–79). London: Routledge.

Parker, I. (2014b). Austerity in the university. *The Psychologist, 27*(45), 236–238.

Parle, S. (2012). How does discrimination affect people with mental illness? *Nursing Times, 108, 28,* 12–14.

Patel, V., Collins, P. Y., Copeland, J., Kakuma, R., Katontoka, S., Lamichhane, J., Naik, S., & Skeen, S. (2011). The movement for global mental health. *The British Journal of Psychiatry, 198*(2), 88–90.

Paul, K. I., & Moser, K. (2009). Unemployment impairs mental health: meta-analyses. *Journal of Vocational Behavior, 74*(3), 264–282.

Peled-Elhanan, N. (2012). *Palestine in Israeli school books: ideology and propaganda in education* (Vol. *82*). London: IB Tauris.

Pells, R. (2017). Sussex University failed duty of care to student assault victim, inquiry finds. *Independent,* 18 January.

Pescosolido, B. A., Perry B. L., Martin J. K., McLeod, J. D., & Jensen, P. S. (2007). Stigmatizing attitudes and beliefs about treatment and psychiatric medications for children with mental illness. *Psychiatric Services, 58*, 613–618.

Pickett, K. E., & Pearl, M. (2001). Multilevel analyses of neighbourhood socio economic context and health outcomes: a critical review. *Journal of Epidemiology & Community Health, 55*(2), 111–122.

Pilgrim, D. (1997). *Psychotherapy and society*. London: Sage.

Place2B (2010). Positive outcomes for children and families: an economic analysis of the Place2B's integrated school-based services for children. Available at www.place2be.org.uk/media/1845/Cost%20Effective%20Positive%20Outcomes%20for%20Children%20and%20Families.pdf (accessed December 2018).

Porter, R. (2002). *Madness: a brief history*. Oxford. Oxford University Press.

Purvis, B., Brandt, R., Rouse, C., Wilfred, V., & Range, L. D. (1988). Students attitudes toward hypothetical chronically and acutely mentally and physically ill individuals. *Psychological Reports, 62*, 627–30.

Quality Care Commission (QCC) (2018). Are we listening? A review of children and young people's mental health services. Available at www.cqc.org.uk/publications/themed-work/are-we-listening-review-children-young-peoples-mental-health-services (accessed December 2018).

Ramos, M. (2013). Psychiatry, authoritarianism, and revolution: the politics of mental illness during military dictatorships in Argentina, 1966–1983. *Bulletin of the History of Medicine, 87*, 250–278.

Rapley, M., Moncrieff, J., & Dillon, J. (Eds.) (2011). *De-medicalizing misery: psychiatry, psychology and the human condition*. New York: Springer.

Read, R., Haslam, N., & Magiano, L. (2013). Prejudice, stigma and 'schizophrenia': the role of bio-genetic ideology. In J. Read & J. Dillon (Eds.), *Models of madness: psychological, social and biological approaches to psychosis* (2nd ed.) (pp. 157–177). London: Routledge.

Reeves, A., McKee, M., & Stuckler, D. (2014). Economic suicides in the Great Recession in Europe and North America. *The British Journal of Psychiatry, 205*(3), 246–247.

Rethink (2011). A user-focused evaluation of IAPT services in London. Report for Commissioning Support for London.Rice-Oxley, M. (2018). It's official: anti-depressants are not snake oil or a conspiracy – they work. Guardian, 21st February.

Richardson, T., Elliot, P., & Roberts, R. (2013). The relationship between personal unsecured debt and mental and physical health: a systematic review and meta-analysis. *Clinical Psychology Review, 33*(8), 1148–1162.

Richardson, T., Elliot, P., Roberts, R., & Jansen, M. (2017). A longitudinal study of financial difficulties and mental health in a national sample of British undergraduate students. *Community Mental Health Journal, 53*(3), 344–352.

Richardson, T., Yeebo, M., Jansen, M., Elliot, P., & Roberts, R. (2018). Financial difficulties and psychosis risk in British undergraduate students: a longitudinal analysis. *Journal of Public Mental Health, 17*(2), 61–68.

Rimke, H. (2018). Sickening institutions: a feminist sociological analysis and critique of religion, medicine, and psychiatry. In J. Kilty & E. Dej (Eds). *Containing madness: gender and 'psy' in institutional contexts*. New York: Palgrave Macmillan.

Rix, J., Nind, M., Simmons, K., & Sheehy, K. (Eds.). (2005). *Policy and power in inclusive education: values into practice*. Hove: Psychology Press.

Rizq, R. (2012a). The perversion of care: psychological therapies in a time of IAPT. *Psychodynamic Practice, 18*(1), 7–24.

Rizq, R. (2012b). The ghost in the machine: IAPT and organizational melancholia. *British Journal of Psychotherapy, 28*(3), 319–335.

Rizq, R. (2017). 'Pre-crime', prevent, and practices of exceptionalism: psychotherapy and the new norm in the NHS. *Psychodynamic Practice, 23*(4), 336–356.

Roberts, B. W., Luo, J., Briley, D. A., Chow, P. I., Su, R., & Hill, P. L. (2017). A systematic review of personality trait change through intervention. *Psychological Bulletin, 143*(2), 117.

Roberts, R. (2015). *Psychology and capitalism*. Winchester. Zero Books.

Roberts, R. (2018). *Capitalism on Campus*. Winchester. Zero Books.

Roberts, R., & Hewer, C. (2015). Memory, 'madness' and conflict: a Laingian perspective. *Memory Studies, 8*(2), 169–182.

Roberts, R., Golding, J., Towell, T., & Weinreb, I. (1999). The effects of students' economic circumstances on British students' mental and physical health. *Journal of American College Health, 48*, 103–109.

Roberts, R., Jones, A., & Sanders, T. (2013) Sex work and students in the UK: providers and purchasers. *Sex Education: Sexuality, Society and Learning, 13*(3), 349–363.

Rogers, A. M. (2017). Star neuroscientist Tom Insel leaves the Google-spawned verily … a startup? *Wired*, 5 November. Available at www.wired.com/2017/05/star-neuroscientist-tom-insel-leaves-google-spawned-verily-startup/ (accessed December 2018).

Rogers, E. (2009). The need for reappraising psychological therapies in the light of IAPT. *The Journal of Mental Health Training, Education and Practice, 4*(1), 19–26.

Rosoux, V., & Anstey, M. (Eds.). (2017). *Negotiating reconciliation in peacemaking: quandaries of relationship building*. New York: Springer.

Roth, A., & Fonagy, P. (2006). What works for whom?: a critical review of psychotherapy research. Guilford Press.

Ryan, F. (2015). Death has become part of Britain's benefits system. *Guardian*, 27 August.

Sagar, T., Jones, D., Tyler, J., Symons, K., & Roberts, R. (2016). Student involvement in the sex industry: findings from the United Kingdom identifying motivations and experiences. *British Journal of Sociology, 67*(4), 697–718.

Salvo, F., Pariente, A., Shakir, S., Robinson, P., Arnaud, M., Thomas, S., +6 others (2016). Sudden cardiac and sudden unexpected death related to antipsychotics: a meta-analysis of observational studies. *Clinical Pharmacology and Therapeutics, 99*, 306–314.

Samadder, R. (2018). Anti-depressants work – but we need to talk too. *Guardian*, 25 February.

Sanders, T., & Hardy, K. (2015). Students selling sex: marketisation, higher education and consumption. *British Journal of Sociology, 36*(5), 747–765.

Savage, M. (2018). Benefit cap leaves poor families with mounting debt, study shows. *Observer*, 3 November.

Schulz, N. (2004). Did antidepressants depress Japan? *New York Times*, 22 August.

Schumacher, E. F. (1973). *Small is beautiful*. London: Vintage.

Scott, M. J. (2018). Improving access to psychological therapies (IAPT) – the need for radical reform. *Journal of Health Psychology*, epub ahead of print, 2 February.

Scott, P. (2017). The end of tuition fees is on the horizon – universities must get ready. *Guardian*, 4 July.

Seabrook, J. (1990). *The myth of the market*. Bideford: Green Books.

Sedgwick, P. (1982). *Psycho politics*. London: Pluto Press.

Selisker, S. (2016). *Human programming: brainwashing, automatons, and American unfreedom*. Minneapolis, MN: University of Minnesota Press.

Sève, L. (1978). *Man in Marxist theory and the psychology of personality*. Sussex. The Harvester Press.

Sharma, R. (2018). Zero hour contract workers triple in UK since 2012 – a quarter of all job growth. *INews* 14 September. https://inews.co.uk/inews-lifestyle/work/zero-hours-contract-uk-statistics-job-growth-since-2012/ (accessed November 2018).

Shaw, T., & Youngblood, D. J. (2010). *Cinematic cold war: the American and Soviet struggle for hearts and minds* (p. 49). Lawrence, KA: University Press of Kansas.

Shildrick, T., & MacDonald, R. (2013). Poverty talk: how people experiencing poverty deny their poverty and why they blame 'the poor'. *The Sociological Review, 61*(2), 285–303.

Silva, C., Ribeiro, J. D., & Joiner, T. E. (2015). Mental disorders and thwarted belongingness, perceived burdensomeness, and acquired capability for suicide. *Psychiatry Research, 226*(1), 316–327.

Skidelsky, R. (2003). *John Maynard Keynes, 1883–1946: economist, philosopher, statesman*. London: Macmillan.

Skidelsky, E., & Skidelsky, R. (2013). *How much is enough? Money and the good life*. London: Penguin.

Skultans, V. (2003). From damaged nerves to masked depression: inevitability and hope in Latvian psychiatric narratives. *Social Science and Medicine, 56*(12): 2421–2431.

Smail, D. (1987). *Taking care: an alternative to therapy*. London. Dent.

Smail, D. J. (2005). *Power, interest and psychology: elements of a social materialist understanding of distress*. Ross-on-Wye: PCCS Books.

Stanford, S., Sharland, E., Heller, N. R., & Warner, J. (2017). *Beyond the risk paradigm in mental health policy and practice*. New York: Macmillan International Higher Education.

Stansfeld, S., & Candy, B. (2006). Psychosocial work environment and mental health – a meta-analytic review. *Scandinavian Journal of Work, Environment & Health, 32*(6), 443–462.

Steptoe, A., Shankar, A., Demakakos, P., & Wardle, J. (2013). Social isolation, loneliness, and mortality. *Proceedings of the National Academy of Sciences, 110*(15), 5797–580.

Stiglitz, J. (2015). The price of inequality: as the stratification of society threatens our future. New York: Norton.

Stonewall (2014). Finding safe spaces. Available at https://stonewallhousing.org/wp-content/uploads/2018/09/FSS_Final_v1.pdf (accessed December 2018).

Streeck, W. (2016). *How will capitalism end?* London: Verso.

Summerfield, D. A. (2017). Western depression is not a universal condition. *British Journal of Psychiatry, 211*, 52.

Swanton, O. (1997). Burden of debt. *Guardian Education*, 3 June, p. iii.

Szasz, T. (1961). *The myth of mental illness*. New York: Harper & Row.

Szasz, T. (2004). *Liberation by oppression: a comparative study of slavery and psychiatry*. London: Transaction.

Szasz, T. (2008). *Psychiatry: the science of lies*. New York: Syracuse University Press.

Telegraph (2012). London Met banned from issuing visas to foreign students. *Telegraph*, 30 August.

Thomas, P., Bracken, P., Cutler, P., Hayward, R., May, R., & Yasmeen, S. (2005). Challenging the globalisation of biomedical psychiatry. *Journal of Public Mental Health*, *4*(3), 23–32.

Thompson, A. (2018) NHS should be run like McDonald's. *Daily Mail*, 28 November.

Thomsen, R. J. (2016). Neoliberal exceptions: racialized debt, crisis, & austerity. Doctoral dissertation, San Francisco State University.

Thomson, I. (2001). Heidegger on ontological education, or: how we become what we are. *Inquiry*, *44*(3), 243–268.

Tiffin, P. A., Pearce, M.S., & Parker, L. (2005). Social mobility over the lifecourse and self-reported mental health at age 50: prospective cohort study. *Journal of Epidemiology & Community Health*, *59*(10), 870–872.

Time to Change (2015). Attitudes to mental illness, 2014 research report. Available at www.time-to-change.org.uk/sites/default/files/Attitudes_to_mental_illness_2014_report_final_0.pdf (accessed January 2019).

Timimi, S. (2010). The McDonaldization of childhood: children's mental health in neo-liberal market cultures. *Transcultural Psychiatry*, *47*(5), 686–706.

Timimi, S. (2013). No more psychiatric labels: campaign to abolish psychiatric diagnostic systems such as ICD and DSM (CAPSID). *Self and Society*, *40*(4), 6–14.

Timimi, S. (2015a). Children and Young People's Improving Access to Psychological Therapies: inspiring innovation or more of the same? *BJPsych Bulletin*, *39*(2), 57–60.

Timimi, S. (2015b). Update on the Improving Access to Psychological Therapies programme in England: author's reply. *BJPsych Bulletin*, *39*(5), 252–253.

Timimi, S. (2018). The diagnosis is correct, but National Institute of Health and Care Excellence guidelines are part of the problem not the solution. *Journal of Health Psychology*, https://doi.org/10.1177/1359105318766139.

Toporek, R. L., Gerstein, L., Fouad, N., & Israel, T. (2006). *Handbook for social justice in counseling psychology: leadership, vision, and action*. London: Sage.

Trades Union Congress (2014). 'Staying Alive': The impact of 'Austerity Cuts' on the LGBT Voluntary and Community Sector (VCS) in England and Wales. Available at www.tuc.org.uk/sites/default/files/StayingAlive_0.pdf. Accessed December 2018.

Truijens, F., Zühlke-van Hulzen, L., & Vanheule, S. (2018). To manualize, or not to manualize: is that still the question? A systematic review of empirical evidence for manual superiority in psychological treatment. *Journal of Clinical Psychology*, epub ahead of print, 28 October.

Tsuang, M. T., Stone, W. S., & Faraone, S. V. (1999). Schizophrenia: a review of genetic studies. *Harvard Review of Psychiatry*, *7*(4), 185–207.

Tucker, A. (2012). Bully U: central planning and higher education. *The Independent Review*, *17*(1), 99–119.

Turner, C. (2017). Investigation into University of Sussex lecturer unearths further reports of alleged harassment and sexual abuse. *Telegraph*, 18 January.

UK Council for Psychotherapy (UKCP) (2015). Addressing the deterioration in public psychotherapy provision. Available at www.ukcp.org.uk/UKCP_Documents/Reports/PublicPsychotherapyProvision-FINAL-WEBsmall.pdf (accessed December 2018).

UN Women (2018) Annual Report 2017–2018. Available at http://annualreport.unwomen.org/en/2018 (accessed January 2019).

United Nations (1948). *Universal declaration of human rights*. Geneva: UN Publications.

United Nations (2018). Statement on visit to the United Kingdom by Professor Philip Alston, United Nations Special Rapporteur on extreme poverty and human rights. Available at www.ohchr.org/Documents/Issues/Poverty/EOM_GB_16Nov2018.pdf (accessed November 2018).

Universities UK (2018). #stepchange: mental health in higher education. Available at www.universitiesuk.ac.uk/stepchange (accessed February 2019).

Vallance, E. (1973). Hiding the hidden curriculum. *Curriculum Theory Network*, *4*, 5–21.

Van der Kolk, B. A. (2014). *The body keeps the score: brain, mind, and body in the healing of trauma*. New York: Penguin.

Van Deurzen, E. (2009). *Everyday mysteries: a handbook of existential psychotherapy*. London: Routledge.

Van Deurzen, E., & Arnold-Baker, C. (2018). *Existential therapy: distinctive features*. London: Routledge.

van Voren, R. (2010). Political abuse of psychiatry: an historical overview. *Schizophrenia Bulletin*, *36*(1), 33–35.

Ventola, C. L. (2011). Direct-to-consumer pharmaceutical advertising: therapeutic or toxic? *Pharmacy and Therapeutics*, *36*(10), 669.

Vos, J. (2016). Working with meaning in life in individuals with a chronic or life-threatening disease: a review of its relevance and the effectiveness of meaning-centered therapies. In P. Russo-Netzer, S. E. Schulenberg, & A. Batthyany (Eds.), *Meaning in positive and existential psychotherapy*. New York: Springer.

Vos, J. (2018). *Meaning in life: an evidence-based handbook for practitioners*. London: Palgrave Macmillan.

Vos, J. (2019). *The economics of meaning in life: the rise and fall of the Capitalist Life Syndrome*. Exeter: University of Exeter Press.

Wahlbeck, K. (2015). Public mental health: the time is ripe for translation of evidence into practice. *World Psychiatry*, *14*(1), 36-42.

Wahlbeck, K., & McDaid, D. (2012). Actions to alleviate the mental health impact of the economic crisis. *World Psychiatry*, *11*(3), 139–145.

Wallerstein, I., Collins, R., Mann, M., Derluguian, G., & Calhoun, C. (2013). *Does capitalism have a future?* Oxford. Oxford University Press.

Watkins, J., Wulaningsih, W., Da Zhou, C., Marshall, D. C., Sylianteng, G. D., Rosa, P. G. D., Miguel, V. A., Raine, R., King, L, P., & Maruthappu, M. (2017). Effects of health and social care spending constraints on mortality in England: a time trend analysis. *BMJ open*, *7*(11), e017722.

Watts, A. (2017). *Psychotherapy east & west*. Novato, CA: New World Library.

Watts, J. (2018). Four-fifths of people believe police austerity cuts have made Britain's streets less safe, poll reveals. *Independent* 10 November. Accessed November 2018.

We Need to Talk Coalition (2017). We still need to talk: a report on access to talking therapies. Available at www.mind.org.uk/media/494424/we-still-need-to-talk_report.pdf (accessed December 2018).

Weale, S. and Batty, D. (2016). University sex abuse report fails to tackle staff attacks on UK students. *Guardian*, 12 October.

Weare, K., & Nind, M. (2011). Mental health promotion and problem prevention in schools: what does the evidence say? *Health promotion international, 26*(suppl_1), i29–i69.

Whitaker, R. (2016). Rising prescriptions, rising disability – is there a link? All-Party Parliamentary Meeting for Prescribed Drug Dependence. Available at http://cepuk.org/2016/05/27/video-now-available-appg-event-link-rising-prescribing-disability/ (accessed December 2018).

Whitaker, R. (2017). Psychiatry under the influence. In J. Davies (Ed.). *The sedated society: the causes and harms of our psychiatric drug epidemic*. London: Palgrave Macmillan.

Whitehead, M., Pennington, A., Orton, L., Nayak, S., Petticrew, M., Sowden, A., & White, M. (2016). How could differences in 'control over destiny lead to socio-economic inequalities in health? A synthesis of theories and pathways in the living environment. *Health & Place, 39*, 51–61.

WHO (1973). *Report of the International Pilot Study of Schizophrenia*, Vol. *1*. Geneva: WHO.

WHO (2000). *Women's mental health: an evidence-based review*. Geneva: WHO. <>

WHO (2001). *World health report: mental health*. Geneva: WHO.

WHO (2003). *Mental health financing*.Geneva: WHO.

WHO (2017). *Mental health atlas*. Geneva: WHO.

WHO (2018). *ICD-11 classifications of mental and behavioural disorder: clinical descriptions and disgnostic guidelines*. Geneva: WHO.

Wilkin, M. (1996). *Initial teacher training: the dialogue of ideology and culture*. London: Falmer Press.

Wilkinson, R., & Pickett, K. (2009). *The spirit level: why equality is better for everyone*. London: Penguin.

Wilkinson, R., & Pickett, K. (2018). *The inner level: how more equal societies reduce stress, restore sanity and improve everyone's wellbeing*. London: Allen Lane.

Wright, N., & Bottery, M. (2002). *Teachers and the state: towards a directed profession*. London: Routledge.

Yarbrough, E. (2018). *Transgender mental health*. Washington, DC: American Psychiatric Association.

YouGov (2016). 'One in four students suffer from mental health problems', 9th August 2016. https://yougov.co.uk/topics/lifestyle/articles-reports/2016/08/09/quarter-britains-students-are-afflicted-mental-hea (accessed November 2018).

Zhang, L. (2017). The rise of therapeutic governing in postsocialist China. *Medical Anthropology, 36*(1), 6–18.

Zizek, S. (2011). *Living in the end times*. London: Verso.

INDEX

Figures and Tables are indicated by page numbers in **bold** print.

www.ingramcontent.com/pod-product-compliance
Lightning Source LLC
Jackson TN
JSHW072034310126
97516JS00004B/14
9781526492203